Mastering Medical Language

Medical Transcription Program
Version 7

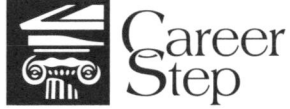

Career Step, LLC
Phone: 801.489.9393
Toll-Free: 800.246.7837
Fax: 801.491.6645
careerstep.com

This text companion contains a snapshot of the online program content converted to a printed format. Please note that the online training program is constantly changing and improving and is always the source of the most up-to-date information.

Product Number: 100502
Generation Date: May 24, 2010

Table of Contents

Unit 1
Introduction

Introduction to Mastering Medical Language

Learning Objective

This module helps the student understand the specialized vocabulary used by healthcare providers and familiarizes the student with a variety of nuances specific to medical language. Specifically, this module will cover word differentiation, abbreviations, plurals, foreign terms, slang, and jargon in medical language.

Suppose someone asked you to read the following list of words and give a brief definition for each: abuse, complex, evening, and live. Sounds simple enough, right? Sure does, unless you consider the following sentences. Look at each of these sentences and read them aloud. You'll see why it is important to read each of them out loud as you continue on in this introduction to Mastering Medical Language.

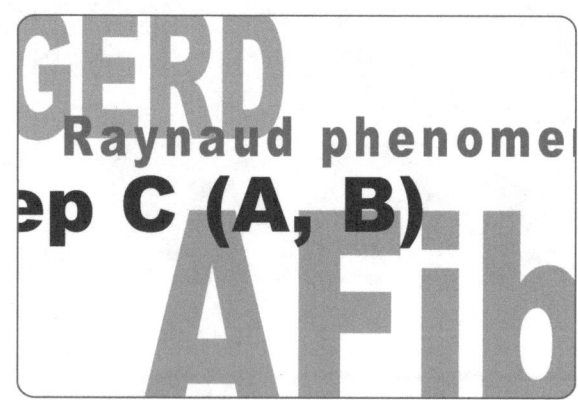

- *His position as a drug **abuse** counselor was a **complex** one. He worked in the **evening** and talked to people **live** in person and on the phone.*

versus

- *While residing in the apartment **complex**, he saw tenants **abuse** their privileges. Once the landlord and the tenants began **evening** out their differences, he continued to **live** there for many years to come.*

As you can see, the mere enunciation of a word changes its meaning dramatically from when the word stands alone on a page. These examples were done using simple words found in everyday use of the English language. When it comes to medical words, imagine the plethora of mistakes that can be made when dealing with the medical language.

As you work through this module on mastering the medical language, keep in mind that the truth is NO ONE can ever truly master every element, facet, and aspect of any language, let alone ever-changing medical words and elements. However, if you are willing to learn some rules, some techniques, and continue with your education both on the job and in your professional pursuits, then you can master one thing: your own destiny!

Medical transcriptionists are translators of a very complex language.

Words can sound alike and look alike but still be vastly different in meaning. For example, you will be learning about the side effect of a medication and how it can affect a person's mood. The difference between the "e" in **effect** (pronounced ee-fekt) and the "a" in **affect** (pronounced ah-fekt) is one you will be studying. These nuances and letter variations can change the entire meaning of a word and ultimately, the diagnosis of a patient. As a medical transcriptionist, you will be hearing the spoken word, but your fingers will translate what those sounds look like on paper. Indeed, medical transcriptionists are translators of a very complex language.

If you were in a supermarket shopping for cabbage, you'd have a mental picture of what a head of cabbage looked like. However, if you heard a doctor order a "CABG" on a patient, you'd be safe to assume that cole slaw should not come to mind. CABG (often pronounced by doctors as "cabbage") actually stands for "coronary artery bypass graft," a surgery within the cardiology realm. As you can see, understanding the spoken word of medicine is but one aspect of becoming a successful medical transcriptionist.

The way a word is abbreviated, singular to plural formations, foreign terminology used in the medical language, slang, and jargon are all components that will be introduced and covered in this module. The more you hear, the more you practice, the more you commit to memory, the more prepared you will be in your journey to become a successful medical transcriptionist!

Unit 2
Word Differentiation

Word Differentiation – Introduction

One of the biggest problems that new medical transcriptionists face is distinguishing between words that, when dictated, sound either identical or so close that the difference is difficult to discern—medical homonyms. A homonym is one of a group of words that share the same spelling or pronunciation (or both) but have different meanings. In this unit we will be focusing specifically on words with the same pronunciation since medical transcription requires documentation of the spoken word. You may remember from the study of prefixes and suffixes terms like inter-/intra- and -phasia/-phagia. There are several examples like these in medical terminology. Your ability to differentiate between the different spellings and meanings will be an important key to your success as a medical transcriptionist.

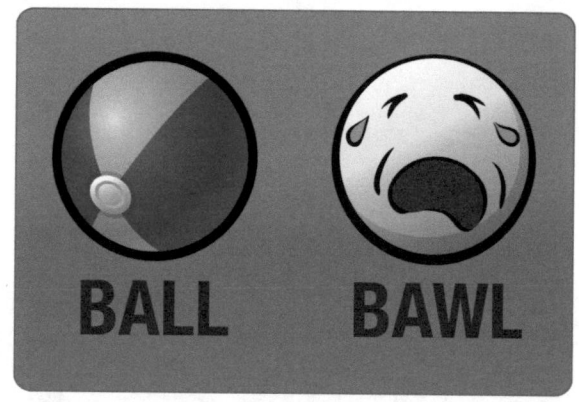

This unit is entirely made up of these difficult words. Pay careful attention to the spelling because a single letter can change the entire meaning of the sentence. Memorize the spellings and respective meanings so that you can consistently use the correct word in a medical report without having to consult a dictionary every time.

Word Differentiation – Lesson 1

1. **accept** versus **except**

   accept – To receive willingly; to agree to.
   She accepted the risks and benefits and agreed to proceed with the treatment.

   except – To take out or leave out; not including; other than.
   There were no complications, except for the excessive bleeding.

2. **adenocyst** versus **adenosis**

   adenocyst – An adenoma in which there is cyst formation.
   The biopsy returned a diagnosis of adenocyst.

   adenosis – Any disease of the glands; the abnormal development or formation of gland tissue.
   The physical examination indicated that there was adenosis in the submandibular gland.

3. **affect** versus **effect**

   affect –
   a) To produce an effect or change on or to exert an influence over (verb).
   b) (As in psychiatry reports) the external expression of emotion (noun).

   a) The digitalis did affect his heart condition. (The "a" is pronounced "uh," as in mud and the stress is on "fect.")
   b) On Mini-Mental State Examination, his affect was flat. (The "a" is pronounced as in cat and the stress is on "af.")

effect –
a) To cause to come into being, to bring about, accomplish, execute (verb).
b) Result, outcome, intent, fulfillment, influence, consequence (noun).

a) A complete cure could be effected if the patient would quit drinking and smoking.
The surgeon's skill was adequate to effect a resolution of the patient's problem.
b) There were no side effects to the medication.
The doctor worked long hours to the effect that he might be of more value to his patients.

4. **affective** versus **effective**

affective – Relating to, arising from, or influencing feelings or emotions.
The patient's affective disorder made him difficult to work with.

effective – Capable of bringing about an effect; exerting positive influence; productive of results, etc.
a) Antibiotics are effective against many bacterial strains.
b) The psychotic nurse's resignation was effective immediately.

5. **afferent** versus **efferent**

afferent – Centripetal, conveying *toward* a center.
There was an afferent loop noted in the colon.

efferent – Centrifugal, conveying *away from* a center.
The efferent nerve was followed.

6. **allusion** versus **elusion** versus **illusion** versus **delusion**

allusion – To refer indirectly or by suggestion.
He made an allusion to an earlier incident.

elusion – Escaping the notice of, an avoidance of, the eluding of something.
The child was a master of elusion whenever his mother was trying to find him.

illusion – A misleading sensory image, such as a mirage; a false interpretation of a real sensory image.
There was no lake in the desert; it was an illusion.

delusion – A false belief that is firmly maintained in spite of proof or evidence to the contrary, as when a patient believes he is Napoleon or Jesus.
In spite of years of treatment, his delusions of grandeur were out of control.

7. **alluding** versus **eluting**

alluding – Referring to in a casual or direct way.
This kind of health insurance is referred to as comprehensive or major medical, alluding to the broad protection offered.

eluting – Removing absorbed material by use of a solvent.
A drug-eluting stent may be used if a vessel is amenable to stent placement.

I. MATCHING.

Match the correct term to the definition. Enter only the letter in the space provided (no punctuation).

1. ____ afferent
2. ____ illusion
3. ____ affect
4. ____ except
5. ____ adenocyst
6. ____ effect
7. ____ accept
8. ____ elusion
9. ____ efferent
10. ____ adenosis
11. ____ effective
12. ____ affective

A. a misleading image
B. to agree to
C. disease of the glands
D. productive of results
E. the avoidance of
F. expression of emotion
G. to leave out
H. arising from emotions
I. away from the center
J. the result or outcome
K. toward the center
L. an adenoma

II. MULTIPLE CHOICE.

Choose the best answer.

1. We were unable to help him to (◯ accept, ◯ except) his mother's death.

2. He seemed to be deeply (◯ affected, ◯ effected) by the loss of his dog.

3. He continued to experience (◯ allusions, ◯ elusions, ◯ delusions) when taking the prescribed medication.

4. We told him to discontinue all medicines (◯ accept, ◯ except) for the Haldol.

5. (◯ Affective, ◯ Effective) use of drugs requires knowledge of their side effects.

6. As it is experimental, all of the side (◯ affects, ◯ effects) are yet unknown.

7. An (◯ afferent, ◯ efferent) loop is a loop formation toward the directional center.

8. He made continued (◯ allusions, ◯ elusions, ◯ illusions) to a traumatic experience while in the war.

9. There was no cyst formation; therefore (◯ adenocyst, ◯ adenosis) was ruled out as possible etiology.

10. There was the inexplicable (◯ allusion, ◯ elusion, ◯ illusion) of the palpated mass on ultrasound.

11. He was diagnosed with a schizo (◯ affective, ◯ effective) disorder.

12. The patient suffered from (◯ adenocyst, ◯ adenosis), or glandular disease, in the parotid gland.

13. Juli kept (◯alluding,◯eluting) to her past history of drug abuse as the major cause for her psychiatric problems.

14. A Taxus drug-(◯alluding,◯eluting) stent was used in the procedure.

Word Differentiation – Lesson 2

1. **aide** versus **aid**

   aide – A person who acts as an assistant, as an aide de camp, nurse's aide, or a teacher's aide. (Note that the term refers to a person.)
   In Alaskan Eskimo villages, most routine healthcare is provided by village health aides.

   aid – Assistance; an assisting device, as a hearing aid, orthotic aid, or aid in transfers. (Note that the term refers to an object.)
   The orthopedic surgeon prescribed a walker as an aid to ambulation.

2. **access** versus **axis**

   access – Capacity to enter or approach; to get at.
   She consented to allow access to her files.

   axis – A line about which a revolving body turns or about which a structure would turn if it did revolve; the second cervical vertebra.
   It was noted to move normally about the axis.

3. **anuresis** versus **enuresis**

   anuresis – Retention of urine in the bladder.
   A Foley catheter was placed secondary to his anuresis.

   enuresis – The involuntary discharge of urine after the age at which urinary control should have been achieved. (Often used in reference to bedwetting.)
   The mother brought the child back for continued enuresis.

4. **acidic** versus **ascitic**

   acidic – Of or pertaining to an acid; acid-forming.
   The urine had an acidic quality to it.

   ascitic –Pertaining to or characterized by ascites: the effusion and accumulation of serous fluid in the abdominal cavity.
   The abdominal cavity was filled with ascitic fluid.

5. **attain** versus **obtain**

   attain – To achieve.
   With all of Carol's experience, she was able to attain her goal of certification.

   obtain – To gain possession of, or to acquire.
   She arrived at the office to obtain a copy of her medical records.

6. **arthrectomy** versus **atherectomy**

   arthrectomy – The excision of a joint.
   He had arthrectomy of his metatarsophalangeal joint.

   atherectomy – The excision of an atheromatous plaque (from an artery).
   There was atherectomy performed of the affected artery.

7. **atonic** versus **atopic** versus **atoxic** versus **atrophic** versus **ectopic**

   atonic – Lacking normal tone or strength.
   Her uterus was markedly atonic.

   atopic – Pertaining to atopy (a genetic predisposition toward the development of hypersensitivity reactions against common environmental antigens=allergies).
   The rash was attributed to atopic causalgia.

   atoxic – Not poisonous; not due to a poison.
   The fluids in his stomach were found to be atoxic.

   atrophic – Pertaining to or characterized by atrophy (wasting away; a diminution in the size of a cell, tissue, organ, or part).
   His muscles were atrophic secondary to his extended hospitalization.

   ectopic – Pertaining to or characterized by displacement or malposition; located away from normal position; arising from abnormal site or tissue.
   She was noted on ultrasound to have a positive ectopic pregnancy.

I. MATCHING.
Match the correct term to the definition.

1. ____ ascitic
2. ____ enuresis
3. ____ axis
4. ____ atherectomy
5. ____ atrophic
6. ____ atoxic
7. ____ acidic
8. ____ ectopic
9. ____ aid
10. ____ anuresis
11. ____ atopic
12. ____ atonic
13. ____ aide
14. ____ access

A. line revolved about
B. acid-forming
C. displaced
D. wasting away
E. retention of urine
F. excision of arterial plaque
G. to get at
H. serous fluid in the abdomen
I. involuntary discharge of urine
J. not poisonous
K. lacking strength
L. pertaining to allergies
M. assisting device
N. person who assists

II. MULTIPLE CHOICE.
Choose the best answer.

1. There was marked (◯ acidic, ◯ ascitic) fluid forming in the abdomen.

2. There was (◯ arthrectomy, ◯ atherectomy) performed of the interphalangeal joint.

3. We worked for three months trying to resolve the child's (◯ anuresis, ◯ enuresis).

4. She was admitted emergently to undergo removal of her (◯ atopic, ◯ atrophic, ◯ atoxic, ◯ ectopic) pregnancy.

5. There was an (◯ acidic, ◯ ascitic) component to the aspirated fluid.

6. She required placement of a Foley catheter secondary to (◯ anuresis, ◯ enuresis).

7. As part of the heart procedure, an (◯ arthrectomy, ◯ atherectomy) was performed of the LIMA.

8. There was (◯ atony, ◯ atopy, ◯ atrophy) of the extremities following the seizure.

9. We were unable to gain (◯ access, ◯ axis) to the mass forming in her abdomen.

10. The drug was determined to be (◯ atopic, ◯ atonic, ◯ atoxic, ◯ atrophic).

11. The patient received (◯aide, ◯aid) at home from a home nursing [12.](◯aide, ◯aid).

13. After she failed to (◯attain, ◯obtain) her goal the third time, she gave up.

14. Dr. Graham (◯attained, ◯obtained) the patient's phone number and called her to the office immediately for her second round of treatment.

Word Differentiation – Lesson 3

1. **avulsion** versus **evulsion**

   avulsion – The forcible tearing away of a body part by trauma or surgery.
   The patient was in a work accident and experienced avulsion of the right index finger.

   evulsion – The act of extracting forcibly.
   Tooth fracture, luxation, evulsion, and socket injury are the main types of dentoalveolar trauma.

2. **aural** versus **oral**

   aural – Pertaining to or perceived by the ear.
   He experienced severe pain when aural stimulus was applied.

   oral – Pertaining to the mouth; taken through or applied in the mouth.
   There were no oral lesions.

3. **bolus** versus **bullous**

   bolus – A rounded mass of food or medicinal preparation ready to swallow, or such a mass passing through the gastrointestinal tract; a mass of pharmaceutical preparation given intravenously for diagnostic purposes.
   She was given a bolus of Pitocin immediately following delivery.

   bullous – Pertaining to or characterized by bullae (a large vesicle, more than 5 mm in circumference, containing serous or seropurulent fluid—also called a bleb or a blister).
   There was bullous disease in the lungs.

4. **brachial** versus **branchial** versus **bronchial**

   brachial – Pertaining to the arm.
   There was brachial swelling noted.

   branchial – Pertaining to or resembling the gills of a fish and having reference to structures in the lateral neck.
   She has a branchial cleft cyst.

   bronchial – Pertaining to one or more bronchi (a subdivision of any of the larger air passages of the lungs).
   There was bronchial wall thickening.

5. **bulbus** versus **bulbous**

> **bulbus** – A rounded mass or enlargement (noun).
> The aortic bulbus was normal.

> **bulbous** – Having the form or nature of a bulb; bearing or arising from a bulb (adjective).
> There was swelling on the bulbous urethra.

6. **callus** versus **callous**

> **callus** – Localized hyperplasia of the horny layer of the epidermis due to pressure or friction (noun).
> The fracture showed callus formation.

> **callous** – Hard, like callus (adjective).
> There was a callous lesion on the surface of the foot.

I. **MATCHING.**
Match the correct term to the definition.

1. ____ brachial
2. ____ bulbous
3. ____ aural
4. ____ bronchial
5. ____ bolus
6. ____ callus
7. ____ oral
8. ____ bullous
9. ____ branchial
10. ____ bulbus
11. ____ callous

A. pertaining to the ear
B. pertaining to the arm
C. medicinal mass
D. hard
E. enlargement
F. characterized by large vesicle
G. resembling fish gills
H. air passage in the lungs
I. pertaining to the mouth
J. localized hyperplasia of the epidermis
K. bulb-like

II. **MULTIPLE CHOICE.**
Choose the best answer.

1. She was given a large (◯ bolus, ◯ bullous) of the medication.

2. A diagnosis of (◯ brachial, ◯ branchial, ◯ bronchial) cleft cyst was made.

3. On (◯ aural, ◯ oral) examination, her tongue was noted to be midline.

4. The anterior urethra consists of the (◯ bulbous, ◯ bulbus) urethra, the pendulous urethra, and the glandular urethra.

5. Extremities examination revealed marked (◯ brachial, ◯ branchial, ◯ bronchial) swelling.

6. The tympanic membranes were noted to be intact on (◯ aural, ◯ oral) examination.

7. On x-ray (◯ callous, ◯ callus) was noted, which indicated healing of the fracture.

8. The lung fields showed marked (◯ bolus, ◯ bullous) changes.

9. The ocular (◯ bulbous, ◯ bulbus) is often referred to as the eye.

10. The patient was given a diagnosis of (◯ brachial, ◯ branchial, ◯ bronchial) pneumonia.

11. While mountain biking, Joe flipped his bike, experiencing a broken wrist and (◯ avulsion, ◯ evulsion) of the middle finger on his left hand.

12. In the accident, the patient experienced 3 molar (◯ avulsions, ◯ evulsions).

Word Differentiation – Lesson 4

1. **canalization** versus **cannulization**

     canalization – The formation of canals, natural or pathologic; the surgical establishment of canals for drainage.
     There was canalization noted throughout the abdominal cavity.

     cannulization – The insertion of a cannula (a tube). (The preferred word is cannulation, but cannulization is used and acceptable.)
     He underwent cannulization in preparation for the operative procedure.

2. **carotid** versus **parotid**

     carotid – Relating to the principal artery of the neck.
     The neck was supple, and no carotid bruits were detected.

     parotid – Situated or occurring near the ear, most commonly as in the parotid gland.
     The parotid gland was normal.

3. **claustrum** versus **colostrum**

     claustrum – The thin layer of grey matter lateral to the external capsule of the lentiform nucleus, separating the nucleus from the white substance of the insula.
     The claustrum was intact.

     colostrum – The thin, yellow, milky fluid secreted by the mammary gland shortly before and a few days after delivery of an infant.
     The baby was receiving colostrum upon breastfeeding.

4. **coaptation** versus **coarctation**

   coaptation – Approximation, as in the edges of a wound or fracture.
   Coaptation of the wound edges was carried out.

   coarctation – A condition of stricture or contraction.
   Coarctation of the aorta was noted.

5. **coarse** versus **course**

   coarse – Not fine; rough/harsh.
   There were coarse crackles noted throughout the lung bases.

   course – Direction of progress; sequence of events; a series of instruction periods; the ground or path over which something moves.
   Her postoperative course was without complications.

I. MATCHING.
Match the correct term to the definition.

1. ___ canalization		A.	neck artery
2. ___ claustrum		B.	approximation
		C.	milky fluid
3. ___ course		D.	rough/harsh
4. ___ coarctation		E.	near the ear
5. ___ colostrum		F.	cannula insertion
6. ___ coarse		G.	contraction
		H.	direction of progress
7. ___ cannulization		I.	layer of grey matter
8. ___ parotid		J.	canal formation
9. ___ coaptation			
10. ___ carotid			

II. MULTIPLE CHOICE.
Choose the best answer.

1. His voice had a (◯ coarse, ◯ course) quality to it.

2. We attempted (◯ canalization, ◯ cannulization) for access into the area.

3. The (◯ carotid, ◯ parotid) gland was noted to be swollen.

4. On examination of the brain, the (◯ claustrum, ◯ colostrum) was within normal limits.

5. (◯ Carotid, ◯ Parotid) pulses were intact.

6. We attempted (⚬ canalization, ⚬ cannulization) to facilitate drainage of the abscess.

7. Throughout the (⚬ coarse, ⚬ course) of hospitalization, her delusional thinking improved.

8. We proceeded with (⚬ coaptation, ⚬ coarctation) of the wound edges.

9. The baby was having trouble extracting the (⚬ claustrum, ⚬ colostrum).

10. There was marked (⚬ coaptation, ⚬ coarctation) of the esophagus.

Word Differentiation – Lesson 5

1. **complement** versus **compliment**

    complement – A quantity needed to make a thing complete; to be complementary to (supplying a defect, making complete, accessory).
    He was given Ensure to complement his diet.

    compliment – An expression of courtesy; a flattering remark **OR** to pay a compliment.
    I complimented him on his choice of words.

2. **conscience** versus **conscious**

    conscience – Consciousness of the moral right and wrong of one's actions.
    He had an extremely guilty conscience.

    conscious – Aware; mentally awake or alert.
    He was not conscious when he was found.

3. **cor** versus **core** versus **corps**

    cor – The muscular organ that maintains the circulation of the blood (the heart).
    Cor: Regular rate and rhythm with no murmurs.
    He was given a diagnosis of cor pulmonale.

    If a patient requests that no heroic measures, such as tubes, cardiopulmonary resuscitation, respirators, etc. be used to prolong his life, he is placed on what is called **NO COR** *status. This is* **ALWAYS** *typed in* **ALL CAPS***.*

    core – The central part of anything.
    A core of tissue was obtained.

    corps – An organized subdivision of a country's military forces.
    He is on active duty with the Marine Corps.

4. **coracoid** versus **choroid**

> **coracoid** – Like a raven's beak (the coracoid process of the scapula).
> There was a small spur noted off the coracoid process.

> **choroid** – The thin, pigmented, vascular coat of the eye, furnishing blood to the retina and conducting arteries and nerves to the anterior structures.
> The choroid plexus is intact.

5. **cytology** versus **sitology**

> **cytology** – The study of cells (their origin, structure, function, and pathology).
> Her cytology exam came back negative.

> **sitology** – The sum of knowledge regarding food, diet, and nutrition.
> The patient's recent sitology is uncertain, as the patient is a poor historian.

I. MATCHING.
Match the correct term to the definition.

1. ____ coracoid	A.	flattering remark
2. ____ cor	B.	beak-shaped
	C.	military division
3. ____ cytology	D.	coating of the eye
4. ____ compliment	E.	awake and alert
5. ____ core	F.	accessory
	G.	knowledge of nutrition
6. ____ conscience	H.	center
7. ____ choroid	I.	the heart
8. ____ complement	J.	moral indicator
9. ____ conscious	K.	study of cells
10. ____ corps		
11. ____ sitology		

II. MULTIPLE CHOICE.
Choose the best answer.

1. He worked for the (◯ Cor, ◯ Core, ◯ Corps) of Engineers.

2. He was given (◯ complementary, ◯ complimentary) antibiotic supplementation.

3. The (◯ coracoid, ◯ choroid) process was intact.

4. He was (◯ conscience, ◯ conscious) on presentation to the emergency room.

5. (◯ Cytology, ◯ Sitology) brought back a diagnosis of squamous cell carcinoma.

6. She received (◯ complements, ◯ compliments) from the nursing staff on her progress.

7. Biopsy yielded a (◯ cor, ◯ core, ◯ corps) of negative tissue.

8. On retinal examination the (◯ coracoid, ◯ choroid) plexus was normal.

9. (◯ Cor, ◯ Core, ◯ Corps) pulmonale is acute strain or hypertrophy of the right heart ventricle.

10. His delusional behavior appears to be the result of nothing more than a guilty (◯ conscience, ◯ conscious).

Word Differentiation – Lesson 6

1. **die** versus **dye**

    die – To stop living.
    He kept saying that he wanted to die.

    dye – Material used for coloring and staining as tests and as therapeutic agents in medicine.
    Dye was injected after the procedure was begun.

2. **discreet** versus **discrete**

    discreet – Showing good judgement; capable of observing prudent silence.
    He was discreet in approaching the subject.

    You will very rarely, if ever, see this spelling used in medical reports.

    discrete – Individually distinct, noncontinuous.
    There were no discrete calcifications.

3. **dysphagia** versus **dysphasia** versus **dysplasia**

    dysphagia – Difficulty swallowing.
    He came in complaining of severe dysphagia.

    dysphasia – Impairment of speech.
    She had dysphasia secondary to a cerebrovascular accident two years ago.

    dysplasia – Abnormality of development; in pathology, alteration in size, shape, and organization of adult cells.
    Dysplasia was noted on biopsy.

4. **echos** versus **echoes**

> **echos** – The plural form of the shortened word echocardiogram.
> His echos all showed T-wave depression.

> **echoes** – The plural form of the word echo—repetition of a sound or the reflection of ultrasonic, radio, and radar waves.
> Cardiac echoes were heard.

5. **elicit** versus **illicit**

> **elicit** – To draw out or forth.
> We could not elicit any further information.

> **illicit** – Not permitted, unlawful.
> He does not take any illicit drugs.

I. **MATCHING.**
Match the correct term to the definition.

1. ___ dye		A.	difficulty swallowing
2. ___ elicit		B.	to stop living
3. ___ dysplasia		C.	plural echocardiogram
4. ___ illicit		D.	individually distinct
5. ___ echoes		E.	impairment of speech
6. ___ die		F.	to draw out
7. ___ dysphasia		G.	illegal
8. ___ discreet		H.	abnormal development
9. ___ dysphagia		I.	material for coloring
10. ___ echos		J.	repetition of sound
11. ___ discrete		K.	showing good judgment

II. **MULTIPLE CHOICE.**
Choose the best answer.

1. There were no (○ discreet, ○ discrete) calcifications.

2. We tried to (○ elicit, ○ illicit) information from her.

3. Following injection of the contrast (○ die, ○ dye) we performed the procedure.

4. The patient had complaints of (○ dysphagia, ○ dysphasia, ○ dysplasia) with all kinds of food.

5. Her (◯ echos, ◯ echoes) were all within normal limits.

6. She drinks a moderate amount of alcohol and is on no (◯ elicit, ◯ illicit) drugs.

7. The patient expressed a wish to (◯ die, ◯ dye).

8. The patient suffered from (◯ dysphagia, ◯ dysphasia, ◯ dysplasia) secondary to her stroke.

9. There were increased (◯ echos, ◯ echoes) on the examination.

10. When talking about his family life, he was generally very (◯ discreet, ◯ discrete).

11. There was marked (◯ dysphagia, ◯ dysphasia, ◯ dysplasia) on pathological examination.

Word Differentiation – Lesson 7

1. **enervation** versus **innervation**

    enervation – Lack of nervous energy; removal of a nerve or a section of a nerve.
    Subsequently he underwent enervation.

    innervation – The distribution or supply of nerves to a part; the supply of nervous energy or of nerve stimulus sent to a part.
    The innervation to the hand was within normal limits.

2. **enterocleisis** versus **enteroclysis**

    enterocleisis – Closure of a wound in the intestine; occlusion of the lumen of the intestine.
    Following thorough inspection, he underwent enterocleisis of the small intestine.

    enteroclysis – The injection of a nutrient or medicinal liquid into the bowel; the introduction of barium directly into the small bowel through a nasogastric tube.
    Following insertion of an NG tube, enteroclysis was undertaken.

3. **exacerbation** versus **exasperation**

    exacerbation – Increase in the severity of a disease or any of its symptoms.
    He had exacerbation of appendicitis symptoms.

    exasperation – Being vexed or irritated.
    She experienced exasperation with the hospital staff.

4. **facial** versus **fascial**

>**facial** – Of or pertaining to the face.
>On HEENT examination there was severe facial swelling.

>**fascial** – Pertaining to or of the nature of a fascia (a sheet or band of fibrous tissue such as lies deep to the skin or forms an investment for muscles and various other organs of the body).
>The cellulitis extended into the fascial layer.

5. **facies** versus **feces**

>**facies** – A term used in anatomical designation of a) the anterior or ventral aspect of the head, forehead to chin inclusive and b) a specific surface of a body structure, part, or organ; the expression or appearance of the face.
>The facies demonstrated fetal alcohol syndrome features.

>**feces** – The excrement discharged from the intestines (poop).
>Feces is scattered throughout the colon.

I. **MATCHING.**
Match the correct term to the definition.

1. ____ exacerbation	A.	pertaining to the face
2. ____ enterocleisis	B.	being irritated
	C.	removal of a nerve
3. ____ enervation	D.	closure of wound
4. ____ innervation	E.	barium injection
5. ____ feces	F.	excrement
	G.	fibrous tissue
6. ____ exasperation	H.	increase of symptoms
7. ____ fascial	I.	expression of face
8. ____ enteroclysis	J.	nerve distribution
9. ____ facies		
10. ____ facial		

II. **MULTIPLE CHOICE.**
Choose the best answer.

1. The colon was packed with (◯ facies, ◯ feces).

2. Following (◯ enervation, ◯ innervation) the wound was closed.

3. The incision was taken down through the (◯ facial, ◯ fascial) plane.

4. The patient experienced an acute (◯ exacerbation, ◯ exasperation) of abdominal pain.

5. Following abdominal exploration, the patient underwent (○ enterocleisis, ○ enteroclysis).

6. (○ Enervation, ○ Innervation) of the foot was within normal limits.

7. The patient has normal (○ facies, ○ feces).

8. Following informed written consent, (○ enterocleisis, ○ enteroclysis) was started.

9. The patient had feelings of (○ exacerbation, ○ exasperation) regarding her progress.

10. The patient experienced a blow to the eye and had severe (○ facial, ○ fascial) swelling.

Review: Lessons 1—7

I. MATCHING.
Match the correct term to the definition. Not all terms will be used.

1. ___	increase in severity of disease	A.	discreet
2. ___	excrement	B.	course
3. ___	a flattering remark	C.	feces
4. ___	moral faculty of the mind	D.	dysphagia
5. ___	localized hyperplasia of epidermis	E.	discrete
6. ___	closure of wound in the intestine	F.	dysphasia
7. ___	impairment of speech	G.	efferent
8. ___	bedwetting	H.	enterocleisis
9. ___	supply of nerves to a part	I.	compliment
10. ___	difficulty swallowing	J.	callus
11. ___	not fine, rough	K.	conscience
12. ___	away from the center	L.	coarse
13. ___	situated or occurring near the ear	M.	exacerbation
14. ___	removal of nerve	N.	accept
15. ___	lacking normal tone	O.	parotid
16. ___	showing good judgement	P.	conscious
17. ___	to refer to indirectly	Q.	innervation
18. ___	insertion of a cannula	R.	enervation
19. ___	to receive willingly	S.	atonic
20. ___	toward the center	T.	callous
		U.	canalization
		V.	cannulization
		W.	anuresis
		X.	allusion
		Y.	enuresis
		Z.	afferent

II. MULTIPLE CHOICE.
Choose the best answer.

1. The patient's low back pain was (○ exasperated, ○ exacerbated) by carrying around her toddler child.

2. The soccer player suffered an orbital rim fracture with severe (○ fascial, ○ facial) swelling.

3. An ultrasound of the heart revealed scant cardiac (○ echoes, ○ echos).

4. The infant was diagnosed with (◯ core, ◯ cor) triloculare, a congential abnormality where the heart has 3 chambers.

5. On mental exam, the patient's (◯ affect, ◯ effect) was normal and mood was euthymic.

6. The patient made no (◯ illusion, ◯ allusion) to what may have caused his panic attacks.

7. A biopsy revealed the breast lump to be sclerosing (◯ adenocyst, ◯ adenosis).

8. Percussion of the abdomen was performed to assess any (◯ ascitic, ◯ acidic) fluid.

9. CT images of the chest revealed (◯ branchial, ◯ bronchial) atresia.

10. The (◯ coarctation, ◯ coaptation) of the wound edges was carried out using staples and Steri-Strips.

Word Differentiation – Lesson 8

1. **fecal** versus **cecal** versus **thecal**

   fecal – Pertaining to or of the nature of feces.
   The patient had a large amount of fecal material scattered throughout the colon.

   cecal – Pertaining to the cecum (any blind pouch or cul-de-sac, usually the first part of the large intestine).
   He underwent ileocecal pouch anastomosis.

   thecal – Pertaining to the theca (an enclosing case or sheath—usually referring to the sac of the spine).
   The mass extended up to the thecal sac.

2. **flexor** versus **flexure**

   flexor – Any muscle that flexes a joint.
   On arthroscopy the flexor tendon was intact.

   flexure – A bending; a bent portion of a structure or organ.
   On colonoscopy exam the hepatic flexure was normal.

3. **fundal** versus **fungal**

   fundal – Pertaining to a fundus (the bottom or base of anything, usually the base of an organ.)
   The mass was located fundal to the liver.

   fungal – Pertaining to or caused by fungus.
   He had a fungal infection.

4. **homogeneous** versus **homogenous**

   homogeneous – Consisting of or composed of similar elements or ingredients; of a uniform quality throughout.
   There was homogeneous echotexture throughout the kidney.

   homogenous – Having a similarity of structure because of descent from a common ancestor.
   The population of Finland is quite homogenous, while the population of the U.S. is not.

5. **hyalin** versus **hyaline**

   hyalin – A translucent albuminoid substance, one of the products of amyloid degeneration; a substance composing the walls of hydatid cysts.
   The cyst wall was composed of hyalin material.

   hyaline – Glassy and transparent, or nearly so.
   The baby was diagnosed with hyaline membrane disease.

I. **MATCHING.**
   Match the correct term to the definition.

   1. ____ fecal
   2. ____ fundal
   3. ____ hyalin
   4. ____ thecal
   5. ____ homogeneous
   6. ____ flexure
   7. ____ homogenous
   8. ____ flexor
   9. ____ cecal
   10. ____ hyaline
   11. ____ fungal

   A. glassy or transparent
   B. sharing a common ancestor
   C. pertaining to the cecum
   D. at the bottom
   E. a muscle flexing a joint
   F. pertaining to excrement
   G. caused by a fungus
   H. albuminoid substance
   I. sac in the spine
   J. a bending
   K. uniform quality

II. **MULTIPLE CHOICE.**
   Choose the best answer.

   1. The cyst was in a (◯fundal, ◯fungal) location.

   2. There was a (◯homogeneous, ◯homogenous) component to the virus.

   3. The hepatic (◯flexor, ◯flexure) was noted to be normal.

   4. There was a (◯fecal, ◯cecal, ◯thecal) residual in the colon.

5. Changes on x-ray examination are probably due to (○hyalin, ○hyaline) membrane disease.

6. Spine x-ray showed a normal (○fecal, ○cecal, ○thecal) sac.

7. The (○flexor, ○flexure) tendon functioned normally.

8. There was (○homogeneous, ○homogenous) echotexture of the liver.

9. The ileo- (○fecal, ○cecal, ○thecal) valve was seen and was normal.

10. He was given medications for presumed (○fundal, ○fungal) infection.

Word Differentiation – Lesson 9

1. **ileum** versus **ilium**

   ileum – The distal portion of the small intestine, extending from the jejunum to the cecum.
   An ileojejunostomy was performed.

   ilium – The expansive superior portion of the hip bone.
   The ilium showed healing, as evidenced by callus formation.

2. **induction** versus **introduction**

   induction – The act or process of inducing or causing to occur—especially the production of anesthesia or unconsciousness by use of the appropriate agents; the appearance of an electric current because of the presence of another electric current.
   The patient underwent Pitocin induction of labor.

   introduction – Leading or bringing in, especially for the first time; to put in.
   Introduction of the Cordis catheter was via the left subclavian approach.

3. **install** versus **instill**
   (or **installation** versus **instillation**)

   install – To establish in an indicated place, condition, or status; to set up for use or service.
   We installed a video camera in the observation room.

   instill – To cause to enter drop by drop; to impart gradually.
   Following instillation of a morphine drip, he was taken off of p.o. medications.

4. **intralocular** versus **intraocular**

intralocular – Within the loculi (small space or cavity) of a structure.
He had intralocular calcifications within the lungs.

intraocular – Within the eye.
The patient underwent intraocular lens implantation.

5. **malleolus** versus **malleus**

malleolus – A rounded process, usually the protuberance on either side of the ankle joint.
The medial malleolus was intact.

malleus – The largest of the auditory ossicles, and the one attached to the membrana tympani.
The cochlea and malleus were entirely normal.

I. **MATCHING.**
Match the correct term to the definition.

1. ___ instill
2. ___ introduction
3. ___ malleolus
4. ___ install
5. ___ intralocular
6. ___ ilium
7. ___ malleus
8. ___ induction
9. ___ ileum
10. ___ intraocular

A. auditory ossicle
B. hip bone
C. within the eye
D. portion of small intestine
E. rounded process
F. inducing anesthesia
G. to establish in place
H. within a cavity
I. enter drop by drop
J. leading or bringing in

II. **MULTIPLE CHOICE.**
Choose the best answer.

1. Following (◯installation, ◯instillation) of contrast, the upper GI examination was done.

2. The lateral (◯malleolus, ◯ malleus) was inspected and found to be entirely within normal limits.

3. The (◯ileum, ◯ilium) was not able to be visualized on the film of the pelvis.

4. She underwent (◯induction, ◯introduction) of general anesthesia.

5. The (◯malleolus, ◯malleus) and vestibule were normal.

6. The (◯ ileo-, ◯ ilio-) cecal valve is normal.

7. The new beds will be (◯ installed, ◯ instilled) in the rooms in one week.

8. There were bullous changes in the (◯ intralocular, ◯ intraocular) areas of the lungs.

9. We will recheck his values following (◯ induction, ◯ introduction) of his new regimen of medicines.

10. The (◯ intralocular, ◯ intraocular) lens was implanted.

Word Differentiation – Lesson 10

1. **median sternotomy** versus **mediastinotomy**

    median sternotomy – The operation of cutting through the midline of the sternum.
    He underwent median sternotomy to begin his heart surgery.

    mediastinotomy – The operation of cutting into the mediastinum (the mass of tissues and organs separating the two pleural sacs).
    X-ray showed evidence of recent mediastinotomy.

2. **mental** versus **omental**

    mental – Pertaining to the mind or chin.
    Mental status is slightly delusional.

    omental – Pertaining to the omentum (a fold of peritoneum extending from the stomach to adjacent organs in the abdominal cavity).
    There was omental obscuration on the abdominal film secondary to poor technique.

3. **metaphysis** versus **metastasis**

    metaphysis – The wider part of the extremity of the shaft of a long bone, adjacent to the epiphyseal disk.
    There was evidence of widening of the metaphysis of the humerus.

    metastasis – The transfer of disease from one organ or part to another not directly connected with it. (Usually referring to malignancy.)
    On bone scan there was evidence of metastasis to the lower spine.

4. **mucous** versus **mucus**

> **mucous** – Pertaining to or resembling mucus; adjectival form of mucus.
> The mucous membranes are normal.
>
> **mucus** – The free slime of the mucous membranes, composed of secretion of the glands, etc.
> On sinus examination there was a great deal of mucus.
>
> *The difference between these two terms is that the -ous ending is an adjectival ending and is used in describing another word (such as membrane). This rule is appropriate for other medical terms, such as viscus/viscous, callus/callous, or bulbus/bulbous, the only difference being the adjectival use.*

5. **osteal** versus **ostial**

> **osteal** – Bony, osseous.
> He had congenital osteal deformities.
>
> **ostial** – Pertaining to an ostium (a door or opening; used to designate an opening into a tubular organ or between two distinct cavities).
> There was ostial thickening noted.

I. **MATCHING.**
   Match the correct term to the definition.

   1. ____ ostial
   2. ____ mucus
   3. ____ metastasis
   4. ____ osteal
   5. ____ mucous
   6. ____ mediastinotomy
   7. ____ metaphysis
   8. ____ median sternotomy
   9. ____ mental
   10. ____ omental

   A. mediastinal operation
   B. pertaining to the mind
   C. a fold of peritoneum (adj.)
   D. part of the long bone
   E. cutting through the sternum
   F. spread of disease
   G. resembling mucus
   H. bony, osseous
   I. free slime
   J. pertaining to a door

II. **MULTIPLE CHOICE.**
    Choose the best answer.

    1. The bony (◯metaphysis, ◯metastasis) of the femur was calcified.

    2. There was a buildup of (◯mucous, ◯mucus) behind the ethmoid sinus.

    3. There was (◯osteal, ◯ostial) thickening of the aorta.

4. A (◯median sternotomy, ◯mediastinotomy) was performed prior to the coronary artery bypass grafting.

5. The (◯mucous, ◯mucus) membranes appeared normal.

6. On (◯mental, ◯omental) status examination there was clarity of thought.

7. The patient's x-ray revealed marked (◯metaphysis, ◯metastasis) to all major organs.

8. The patient had (◯ osteal, ◯ostial) pain in her ankles.

9. A (◯median sternotomy, ◯mediastinotomy) was performed secondary to metastasis to the mediastinum.

10. The (◯mental, ◯omentum) was noted to be intact.

Word Differentiation – Lesson 11

1. **parental** versus **parenteral**

    parental – Pertaining to one that begets offspring.
    Following informed parental consent, the ORIF was performed on the child.

    parenteral – Not through the alimentary canal, but rather by injection through some other route, such as subcutaneous, intramuscular, intravenous, etc.
    The patient was begun on total parenteral nutrition.

2. **perineal** versus **peroneal**

    perineal – Pertaining to the perineum (the region between the thighs, bounded in the male by the scrotum and anus and in the female by the vulva and anus).
    The patient experienced marked perineal irritation during intercourse.

    peroneal – Pertaining to the fibula or to the outer side of the leg.
    The peroneal ligament was found to be slightly torn.

3. **perineum** versus **peritoneum**

    perineum – (see above)—the region between the thighs.
    On digital examination the perineum was found to be normal.

    peritoneum – The serous membrane lining the abdominopelvic walls.
    On exploration of the abdomen, the peritoneum was noted to be intact.

4. **plain** versus **plane**

> **plain** – Free of extraneous matter; simple, uncomplicated; lacking beauty.
> On plain film examination of the abdomen there was a mass noted behind the liver.

> **plane** – A surface such that a straight line connecting any two of its points lies wholly in the surface.
> Films were taken in the sagittal plane.

5. **precede(d)** versus **proceed(ed)**

> **precede** – To be, go, or come ahead or in front of.
> Preceding the instillation of general anesthesia, the patient's vital signs were recorded.

> **proceed** – To go on in an orderly way; continue
> We proceeded to carry the incision down through the subcutaneous layer.

I. **MATCHING.**
    Match the correct term to the definition.

1. ____ plain
2. ____ proceed
3. ____ peritoneum
4. ____ peroneal
5. ____ precede
6. ____ perineum
7. ____ plane
8. ____ parenteral
9. ____ perineal
10. ____ parental

A. area between the thighs
B. pertaining to parents
C. to go in front of
D. simple
E. injection by alternate route
F. pertaining to the perineum
G. continue
H. fibular
I. serous membrane/abdomen
J. a straight surface

II. **MULTIPLE CHOICE.**
    Choose the best answer.

1. During surgical exploration of the abdominal cavity, the (○perineum, ○peritoneum) was noted to be normal.

2. We decided to (○precede, ○proceed) with his physical therapy.

3. The (○perineal, ○peroneal) ligament was torn.

4. We followed the normal (○plain, ○plane) of dissection.

5. He was begun on total (○parental, ○parenteral) nutrition.

6. A (◯plain, ◯plane) film was taken of the head.

7. Consent (◯preceded, ◯proceeded) hospitalization.

8. The youth is strongly in need of (◯parental, ◯parenteral) guidance.

9. Her (◯perineum, ◯peroneum) was torn during intercourse.

Word Differentiation – Lesson 12

1. **perfusion** versus **profusion** versus **protrusion**

    perfusion – The act of pouring over or through, especially the passage of fluid through the vessels of a specific organ.
    There was normal perfusion of the lungs.

    profusion – Abundance, pouring forth with great liberality.
    There was a profusion of mucous discharge from her nose.

    protrusion – The state of being thrust forward.
    There was protrusion of the orthopedic nail through the skin.

2. **prostate** versus **prostrate**

    prostate – A gland in the male that surrounds the neck of the bladder and the urethra.
    Genitourinary exam revealed a normal sized prostate.

    prostrate – Extended in a horizontal position.
    The patient was prostrate upon the ground when the ambulance arrived.

3. **prostatic** versus **prosthetic**

    prostatic – Related to the prostate.
    His benign prostatic hypertrophy exhibited the usual symptoms.

    prosthetic – Referring to an artificial limb or other artificial structure in the body.
    He had a prosthetic heart valve.

4. **reflex** versus **reflux**

    reflex – A reflected action or movement; the sum total of any particular involuntary activity.
    Deep tendon reflexes were 2+ and normal.

    reflux – A backward or return flow.
    The patient presented for symptoms of reflux esophagitis.

5. **regimen** versus **regiment**

   regimen – A strictly regulated scheme of diet, exercise, or other activity designed to achieve certain ends.
   His regimen consisted of Zantac and Diabinese.

   regiment – A military unit.
   His regiment was stationed in Saigon.

6. **residence** versus **residents** versus **resonance**

   residence – The place where one lives.
   His place of residence is 1200 E. University Ave, Nowhere, Maine.

   residents – Those who live in a place; physicians serving in residency.
   The examination was performed by the residents on call.

   resonance – The prolongation and intensification of sound produced by the transmission of its vibrations to a cavity; a vocal sound as heard in auscultation.
   The lungs were normal on resonance exam.

I. **MATCHING.**
    Match the correct term to the definition.

1. ___ prostate		A.	relating to a male gland
2. ___ profusion		B.	male gland
		C.	involuntary action
3. ___ resonance		D.	lying horizontal
4. ___ perfusion		E.	abundance
5. ___ regimen		F.	military unit
		G.	artificial part
6. ___ reflex		H.	where one lives
7. ___ residence		I.	pouring over or through
8. ___ reflux		J.	backward flow
		K.	strictly regulated activity
9. ___ prostrate		L.	being thrust forward
10. ___ regiment		M.	vocal sound
11. ___ protrusion			
12. ___ prosthetic			
13. ___ prostatic			

II. MULTIPLE CHOICE.
Choose the best answer.

1. During the (◯ perfusion, ◯ profusion, ◯ protrusion) scan, a health care provider injects radioactive albumin into the patient's vein.

2. A strict (◯ regimen, ◯ regiment) of antibiotics was started.

3. The patient was found on biopsy to have (◯ prostate, ◯ prostrate) cancer.

4. There were normal (◯ reflexes, ◯ refluxes) exhibited throughout the extremities.

5. There was (◯ perfusion, ◯ profusion, ◯ protrusion) of the intestine through the abdominal wall.

6. The patient should remain (◯ prostate, ◯ prostrate) for at least two weeks.

7. There were three (◯ residence, ◯ residents, ◯ resonance) assigned to his care.

8. The PSA was negative for any recurrent (◯ prostatic, ◯ prosthetic) disease.

9. There was a normal (◯ residence, ◯ residents, ◯ resonance) of sound.

10. He was checked for sandfly disease secondary to his (◯ regimen, ◯ regiment) being assigned to the Persian Gulf.

11. The patient was fitted with a (◯ prostatic, ◯ prosthetic) device.

12. The patient had symptoms of (◯ reflex, ◯ reflux) esophagitis.

Word Differentiation – Lesson 13

1. **root** versus **route**

   root – The lowermost part, or a structure by which something is firmly attached.
   The aortic root was identified and appeared normal.

   route – Channel; a line of travel.
   The catheter was passed through the internal jugular route.

2. **Scarpa's** versus **scarpus**

   Scarpa's – (Scarpa's fascia) is the deep membranous layer of subcutaneous abdominal fascia.
   An incision was made lateral to Scarpa's fascia.

   scarpus – This is not a real word; however, new medical transcriptionists will often type it anyway. Make sure you know that the correct word is Scarpa's.

3. **silicon** versus **silicone**

    silicon – A nonmetallic element occurring in nature.
    There was a heavy concentration of silicon in the dirt.

    silicone – Any organic compound in which all or part of the carbon has been replaced by silicon.
    The patient has had a previous silicone breast implant.

4. **sight** versus **site**

    sight – The process, function, or power of seeing.
    The patient has very poor sight in his left eye.

    site – A place, position, or locus.
    There was cellulitis at the site of the patient's previous incision.

5. **track** versus **tracked** versus **tract**

    track – Path, route; the path along which something moves, or the mark left by its movement.
    The patient is on the right track for a full recovery.

    tracked – Past tense of track.
    We tracked the progress of the disease.

    tract – A region, usually one of some length; specifically a collection of nerve fibers or a number of organs, arranged in a series, serving a common function.
    There was no thickening of the fistulous tract.

I. **MATCHING.**
Match the correct term to the definition.

1. ____ silicone	A.	the lowermost portion
2. ____ sight	B.	nonmetallic element
3. ____ scarpus	C.	a location
4. ____ site	D.	path
5. ____ track	E.	channel
6. ____ Scarpa's	F.	organic compound
7. ____ tract	G.	seeing
8. ____ root	H.	a region
9. ____ silicon	I.	deep membranous layer
10. ____ route	J.	not a real word

II. MULTIPLE CHOICE.
Choose the best answer.

1. The catheter was entered via left subclavian (◯root, ◯ route).

2. The (◯sight, ◯site) of the patient's scar was severely edematous.

3. A cyst was noted just inferior to (◯Scarpa's, ◯scarpus) fascia.

4. The patient had recent (◯silicon, ◯silicone) breast implantation performed.

5. The patient's (◯sight, ◯site) was very poor secondary to cataracts.

6. The aortic (◯root, ◯ route) appeared within normal limits.

7. The sinus (◯track, ◯tracked, ◯tract) was clear of obstruction.

8. The compound was tested for (◯silicon, ◯silicone).

9. Laboratory values were (◯track, ◯tracked, ◯tract) throughout the hospital course.

Word Differentiation – Lesson 14

1. **uncal** versus **ungual** versus **lingual**

   uncal – Pertaining to the uncus (any hook-shaped structure; the medially curved anterior end of the parahippocampal gyrus).
   There is narrowing of the uncovertebral joint.

   ungual – Pertaining to the nails (fingernails and toenails).
   There was subungual swelling noted on musculoskeletal examination.

   lingual – Pertaining to or towards the tongue.
   The patient was instructed to take sublingual nitroglycerin p.r.n.

2. **vertex** versus **vortex**

   vertex – Summit or top; the top or crown of the head.
   Obstetrical ultrasound showed the fetus to be in vertex presentation.

   vortex – A whorled arrangement, design, or pattern, as of muscle fibers, or of the ridges or hairs on the skin.
   The patient had a vortex pattern on the ends of his fingers.

3. **viscus** versus **viscous**

> **viscus** – (Plural is viscera.) A large internal organ of the body. Especially one located in the great cavity of the trunk. (noun)
> The heart is a viscus, as is the liver, spleen, or gallbladder.
>
> **viscous** – Descriptive word for a liquid that is thick and slow-flowing.
> Viscous lidocaine was given for anesthesia.

4. **waist** versus **waste**

> **waist** – The portion of the body between the thorax and the hips; a part resembling the human waist, especially in narrowness or central position.
> The waist of the scaphoid was intact.
>
> **waste** – Gradual loss, decay, or diminution of bulk; damaged, defective, or superfluous material; refuse.
> There was wasting away of his muscle tissue.

5. **Xanax** versus **Zantac**

> **Xanax** – A drug used as a muscle relaxant and for anxiety disorders.
> The patient was prescribed Xanax for inability to sleep.
>
> **Zantac** – A drug used in the treatment of ulcers.
> The patient was put on Zantac and Milk of Magnesia.

I. **MATCHING.**
   Match the correct term to the definition.

1. ____ lingual		A. between the chest and hips
2. ____ vertex		B. used for anxiety
3. ____ uncal		C. hook-shaped (adj.)
4. ____ Zantac		D. summit or top
5. ____ viscous		E. used for ulcers
6. ____ ungual		F. gradual loss or decay
7. ____ waist		G. towards the tongue
8. ____ Xanax		H. a whorled design
9. ____ waste		I. pertaining to the nails
10. ____ vortex		J. large organ
11. ____ viscus		K. thick and slow-flowing

II. MULTIPLE CHOICE.
Choose the best answer.

1. The skin had a (○ vertex, ○ vortex) pattern.

2. (○ Xanax, ○ Zantac) was prescribed for peptic ulcer disease.

3. The patient had her temperature taken (○ subuncally, ○ subungually, ○ sublingually).

4. Amniotic fluid is normal and the fetus is in a (○ vertex, ○ vortex) presentation.

5. The patient had gradual (○ waisting, ○ wasting) away of his mental capacities.

6. The patient was placed on (○ Xanax, ○ Zantac) following her violent rage.

7. A pin was jammed into the (○ subuncal, ○ subungual, ○ sublingual) region and it necessitated the removal of the nail.

8. She is unable to bend at the (○ waist, ○ waste).

9. The (○ uncal, ○ ungual) structure was normal on the cervical spine x-ray.

10. During surgery care was taken to avoid damage to any (○ viscus, ○ viscous).

11. Upon cutting into the brain during the autopsy, a (○ viscus, ○ viscous) fluid oozed out.

Review: Lessons 8—14

I. **MATCHING.**
   Match the correct term to the definition. Not all terms will be used.

1. ___ within the eye		A. ostial
2. ___ resembling glass in transparency or translucency		B. flexor
		C. hyalin
3. ___ physicians serving in residency		D. perfusion
4. ___ a place or position		E. site
5. ___ pertaining to the nails		F. proceed
6. ___ pertaining to the outer side of the leg		G. intraocular
7. ___ extended in horizontal position		H. residents
8. ___ a muscle that flexes a joint		I. flexure
9. ___ abundance, large quantity		J. prostrate
		K. plain
10. ___ simple, uncomplicated		L. perineal
11. ___ male gland		M. osteal
12. ___ process of seeing		N. reflux
13. ___ the place where one lives		O. profusion
14. ___ pertaining to a structure that is long, thin, and curved		P. ungual
		Q. residence
15. ___ to continue in an orderly way		R. hyaline
16. ___ bony, osseous.		S. uncal
		T. track
17. ___ path, route		U. prostate
18. ___ the act of pouring over or through		V. intralocular
		W. tract
19. ___ pertaining to the region between the thighs		X. plane
20. ___ a backward or return flow		Y. peroneal
		Z. sight

II. **MULTIPLE CHOICE.**
   Choose the best answer.

1. The (○ sight, ○ site) of the wound was cleaned and dressed.

2. His blood sugar levels were (○ tract, ○ tracked) over the course of 24 hours.

3. The wound drained purulent and (○ viscous, ○ viscus) material.

4. The bone (◯ protrusion, ◯ perfusion) through the skin indicated an open fracture.

5. The patient was started on a low-salt (◯ regimen, ◯ regiment).

6. Informed consent (◯ preceded, ◯ proceeded) the procedure.

7. The (◯ plane, ◯ plain) film of the ankle revealed no fracture.

8. His nose drained clear (◯ mucus, ◯ mucous).

9. The patient is being seen for a suspected (◯ fungal, ◯ fundal) infection on his foot.

10. There was (◯ osteal, ◯ ostial) thickening noted.

Unit 3
Abbreviations

Abbreviations – Introduction

In medical reports, there is a lot of repetition. All over the world, people acquire the same diseases and syndromes, have the same body parts and symptoms, and have the same tests performed with similar laboratory values. As a result, many of these terms and phrases have come to be known by their respective abbreviations. This speeds up dictation, and the abbreviations have become so commonly used among medical personnel that the meanings are universally known. You will be a more productive and efficient medical transcriptionist if you are familiar with the common abbreviations. Be aware that the abbreviations you will study in this material are not *all* of the abbreviations used in medical dictation, although you

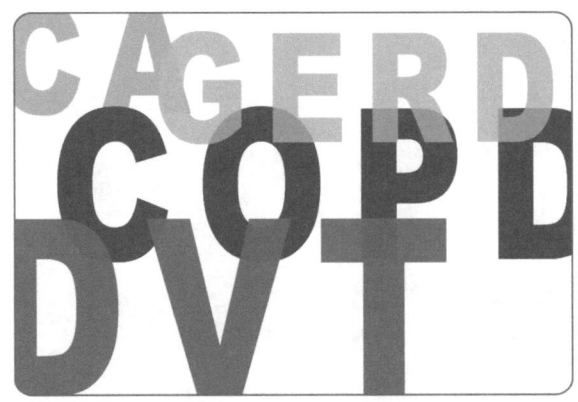

will be exposed to comprehensive categories of abbreviations. Additionally, many abbreviations have more than one correct expansion, and a good abbreviations reference will go a long way in helping determine what the correct expansion is for a particular abbreviation. You will be exposed to additional abbreviations as you work through the course, and to still others as you master medical transcription in the workplace.

The spoken word is often easy to misunderstand, especially when it is being said fast or mumbled into dictation equipment. If you are unfamiliar with the abbreviations from the outset, it is extremely difficult to differentiate between certain letters; for example, an *S* and an *F* or a *D* and a *T*. Therefore, while you are doing the following exercises, you should say the configuration of letters out loud a few times to familiarize yourself with the sound. When you hear the same abbreviation in an actual report, this will make it easier to understand and recognize.

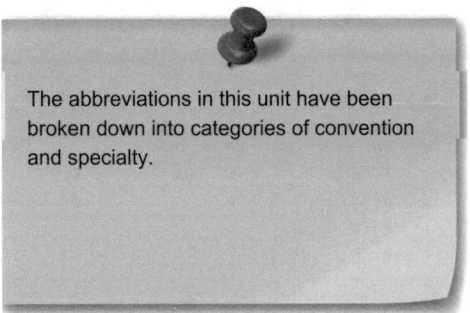

The abbreviations in this unit have been broken down into categories of convention and specialty.

Often hospitals and doctors will require you to expand dictated abbreviations. That means that not only do you need to be able to identify what letters are being said, but also what they stand for. The more of these you are able to identify without having to look them up, the faster and more efficient a transcriptist you are.

The most common method of dictating entails simply listing the letters in the appropriate order, such as C-A-D, saying each letter individually. Another way of dictating an abbreviation is to pronounce the abbreviation as a word, such as "gerd" (sounds like herd) for G-E-R-D. This is rare, and you will be introduced to it as it occurs.

The abbreviations unit has been broken down into categories of convention and specialty. This is to help you not only associate the letters themselves with their respective meanings, but also with their appropriate context. Pay attention to the classification into which each abbreviation fits. Learn these abbreviations thoroughly and what they stand for.

Diseases and Syndromes – Lesson 1

The abbreviations for syndromes and diseases are both the most extensive and the most commonly used abbreviations, aside perhaps from those used in laboratory data. Many of these abbreviations will be repeated in other categories within this unit. This is done by design—to give you repeated exposure to some of the most commonly used abbreviations. It would be a good idea to memorize these abbreviations.

The diseases that tend to be abbreviated are the ones that affect the largest number of people. You will see these often in diagnosis lists and histories. If you are administered a test by a potential employer who requires you to expand abbreviations, that test will likely be taken primarily from the following lists.

I. ENTER ABBREVIATIONS.
Enter the abbreviation and what it stands for.

AAA: abdominal aortic aneurysm
Upon exploration of the abdomen, no AAA was noted.

    1. _____ (Abbreviation)

    2. _____

This particular abbreviation will often be dictated "triple A," but should always be typed AAA.

AIDS: acquired immune deficiency syndrome
The patient has AIDS, stage V.

    3. _____ (Abbreviation)

    4. _____

AIDS is almost exclusively pronounced as the word its letters spell.

ALL: acute lymphocytic leukemia (acute lymphoblastic leukemia)
The patient has advanced ALL.

    5. _____ (Abbreviation)

    6. _____

    7. _____

ARDS: adult respiratory distress syndrome
She has known ARDS, with a long history of smoking.

    8. _____ (Abbreviation)

    9. _____

BPH: benign prostatic hypertrophy
On biopsy, he was found to have BPH.

    10. _____ (Abbreviation)

    11. _____

Benign prostatic hyperplasia is also an acceptable expansion of BPH.

II. FILL IN THE BLANK.
Some spaces may require more than one word. Be sure to provide the complete answer. For any question that may have more than one appropriate answer, just choose one.

1. She was admitted with a known history of adult _____ distress
   2. _____ .

3. He has known _____ immune ⁴· _____ syndrome.

5. On prostate exam he was found to have benign prostatic _____ .

6. Acute _____ leukemia was diagnosed three months ago.

7. She has an abdominal aortic _____ .

III. FILL IN THE BLANK.
Expand the following abbreviations. For any abbreviation that has more than one expansion, just choose one that is appropriate for this lesson.

1. BPH _____   2. AIDS _____

3. AAA _____   4. ALL _____

5. ARDS _____

Diseases and Syndromes – Lesson 2

I. ENTER ABBREVIATIONS.
Enter the abbreviation and what it stands for.

CA: cancer or carcinoma
The patient has a history of CA of the liver.

1. _____ (Abbreviation)

2. _____

CF: cystic fibrosis
He was hospitalized twice for his CF.

3. _____ (Abbreviation)

4. _____

CHF: congestive heart failure
He presented with CHF.

5. _____ (Abbreviation)

6. _____

CMV: cytomegalovirus
She was diagnosed with CMV.

    7. _____ (Abbreviation)

    8. _____

COPD: chronic obstructive pulmonary disease
He has a history of COPD.

    9. _____ (Abbreviation)

  10. _____

CVA: cerebrovascular accident
The patient presented to the emergency room with symptoms of CVA.

  11. _____ (Abbreviation)

  12. _____

CVA also stands for costovertebral angle and is frequently dictated in the physical exam portion of a report. Make sure, by careful attention to context, that you use the correct one.

II. **FILL IN THE BLANK.**
Some spaces may require more than one word. Be sure to provide the complete answer. For any question that may have more than one appropriate answer, just choose one.

  1. She has adeno _____ of the kidneys.

  2. The patient has _____ pulmonary disease.

  3. He presented with _____ heart failure.

  4. A diagnosis of _____ fibrosis was made.

  5. On testing he was found to have suffered a _____ accident.

  6. Cyto_____ is his primary diagnosis.

III. **FILL IN THE BLANK.**
Expand the following abbreviations. For any abbreviation that has more than one expansion, just choose one that is appropriate for this lesson.

1. CMV_____   2. COPD_____

3. CHF_____   4. CA_____

5. CVA_____   6. CF_____

I. **ENTER ABBREVIATIONS.**
   Enter the abbreviation and what it stands for.

   DISH: diffuse idiopathic skeletal hyperostosis
   On skeletal survey he was found to have DISH.

   1. _____ (Abbreviation)

   2. _____

   The introduction to this chapter stated that there were two primary ways of dictating abbreviations. You have already had several examples of the first, namely, saying each individual letter. This is an example of the second method of dictating abbreviations. DISH is almost exclusively pronounced as the word its letters spell (dish—as in plate or bowl).

   DJD: degenerative joint disease
   He has DJD of the acromioclavicular joint.

   3. _____ (Abbreviation)

   4. _____

   DM: diabetes mellitus
   The patient's blood sugars are high, consistent with a history of DM.

   5. _____ (Abbreviation)

   6. _____

   DVT: deep venous thrombosis (deep vein thrombosis)
   The patient is on Coumadin for DVT.

   7. _____ (Abbreviation)

   8. _____

   FCD: fibrocystic disease
   On mammogram the breasts show a pattern consistent with FCD.

   9. _____ (Abbreviation)

   10. _____

II. **FILL IN THE BLANK.**
   Some spaces may require more than one word. Be sure to provide the complete answer. For any question that may have more than one appropriate answer, just choose one.

   1. X-ray shows evidence of diffuse _____ skeletal 2. _____.

   3. Ultrasound of the leg showed deep venous _____.

4. _____ disease was noted on mammogram.

5. The patient takes insulin for her diabetes _____.

6. He has a history of _____ joint disease.

III. **FILL IN THE BLANK.**
Expand the following abbreviations. For any abbreviation that has more than one expansion, just choose one that is appropriate for this lesson.

1. DVT_____   2. DM_____

3. DJD_____   4. DISH_____

5. FCD_____

Diseases and Syndromes – Lesson 4

I. **ENTER ABBREVIATIONS.**
Enter the abbreviation and what it stands for.

GERD: gastroesophageal reflux disease
GI consulted and gave a diagnosis of GERD.

1. _____ (Abbreviation)

2. _____

HMD: hyaline membrane disease
The baby's ultrasound is consistent with HMD.

3. _____ (Abbreviation)

4. _____

HNP: herniated nucleus pulposus
He has HNP noted at L4-5.

5. _____ (Abbreviation)

6. _____

IDDM: insulin-dependent diabetes mellitus
His IDDM was poorly controlled.

7. _____ (Abbreviation)

8. _____

ILD: interstitial lung disease
Chest x-ray confirmed ILD.

    9. _____ (Abbreviation)

    10. _____

II. **FILL IN THE BLANK.**
Some spaces may require more than one word. Be sure to provide the complete answer. For any question that may have more than one appropriate answer, just choose one.

    1. Gastroesophageal _____ disease was noted.

    2. _____ nucleus 3. _____ at C3-4.

    4. _____ lung disease is present.

    5. She takes NPH for her _____ diabetes mellitus.

    6. Her _____ membrane disease is a result of prematurity.

III. **FILL IN THE BLANK.**
Expand the following abbreviations. For any abbreviation that has more than one expansion, just choose one that is appropriate for this lesson

1. HMD_____   2. GERD_____

3. IDDM_____   4. HNP_____

5. ILD_____

Diseases and Syndromes – Lesson 5

I. **ENTER ABBREVIATIONS.**
Enter the abbreviation and what it stands for.

MS: multiple sclerosis
Her MS precluded general anesthetic.

    1. _____ (Abbreviation)

    2. _____

PTSD: post-traumatic stress disorder
The veteran suffered from PTSD.

    3. _____ (Abbreviation)

    4. _____

RA: rheumatoid arthritis
Findings compatible with rheumatoid arthritis.

   5. _____ (Abbreviation)

   6. _____

RSD: reflex sympathetic dystrophy
The patient has known RSD.

   7. _____ (Abbreviation)

   8. _____

RSV: respiratory syncytial virus
He was diagnosed with RSV pneumonia.

   9. _____ (Abbreviation)

  10. _____

II. FILL IN THE BLANK.
Some spaces may require more than one word. Be sure to provide the complete answer. For any question that may have more than one appropriate answer, just choose one.

   1. She was diagnosed with multiple _____ .

   2. Severe _____ arthritis can cause deformity of the joints.

   3. The patient has a history of reflex sympathetic _____ .

   4. Respiratory _____ virus was the primary diagnosis.

   5. _____ stress disorder was evident.

III. FILL IN THE BLANK.
Expand the following abbreviations. For any abbreviation that has more than one expansion, just choose one that is appropriate for this lesson.

1. MS_____   2. PTSD_____

3. RSV_____   4. RA_____

5. RSD_____

Diseases and Syndromes – Lesson 6

I. ENTER ABBREVIATIONS.
Enter the abbreviation and what it stands for.

SIDS: sudden infant death syndrome
The autopsy was negative, suggesting a diagnosis of SIDS.

1. _____ (Abbreviation)

2. _____

SIDS is almost exclusively pronounced as the word its letters spell.

SLE: systemic lupus erythematosus
The symptoms point to a diagnosis of SLE.

3. _____ (Abbreviation)

4. _____

TIA: transient ischemic attack
The patient has a history of chronic TIAs.

5. _____ (Abbreviation)

6. _____

URI: upper respiratory infection
With negative strep, URI is the most likely diagnosis.

7. _____ (Abbreviation)

8. _____

UTI: urinary tract infection
She has a long history of UTIs.

9. _____ (Abbreviation)

10. _____

II. FILL IN THE BLANK.
Some spaces may require more than one word. Be sure to provide the complete answer. For any question that may have more than one appropriate answer, just choose one.

1. He presented to the ER last week with an upper _____ infection.

2. Cause of death was _____ lupus 3. _____.

4. He was admitted for a transient _____.

5. She was given antibiotics for a _____ tract [6.] _____ .

7. The baby died of _____ infant death [8.] _____ .

III. **FILL IN THE BLANK.**
Expand the following abbreviations. For any abbreviation that has more than one expansion, just choose one that is appropriate for this lesson.

1. TIA_____   2. UTI_____

3. SLE_____   4. URI_____

5. SIDS_____

Review: Diseases and Syndromes

I. **FILL IN THE BLANK.**
Some spaces may require more than one word. Be sure to provide the complete answer. For any question that may have more than one appropriate answer, just choose one.

1. degenerative _____ disease

2. _____ vascular accident

3. chronic _____ disease

4. sudden infant _____

5. _____ ischemic attack

6. congestive heart _____

7. upper _____ infection

8. deep _____

9. _____ tract infection

10. diffuse _____ hyperostosis

cerebro
death syndrome
failure
idiopathic skeletal
joint
obstructive pulmonary
respiratory
transient
urinary
venous thrombosis

II. MATCHING.

Match the word or word part to the abbreviation expansion. You may use each answer more than once, or not at all.

1. ____ UTI – urinary tract _____

2. ____ RA – rheumatoid _____

3. ____ CMV – _____ virus

4. ____ DM – diabetes _____

5. ____ HMD – hyaline _____ disease

6. ____ RSV – respiratory _____ virus

7. ____ PTSD – post-traumatic _____ disorder

8. ____ DVT – deep venous _____

9. ____ CA – _____

10. ____ TIA – _____ ischemic attack

A. cytomegalo
B. syncytial
C. thrombosis
D. carcinoma
E. transient
F. mellitus
G. infection
H. arthritis
I. stress
J. membrane

III. MULTIPLE CHOICE.

Choose the correct word or word part for the abbreviation expansion.

1. SLE – systemic lupus (◯ erythematous, ◯ erythematosus)

2. FCD – fibro (◯ chronic, ◯ cystic) disease

3. RSD – reflex (◯ sympathetic, ◯ systemic) dystrophy

4. HNP – herniated nucleus (◯ pulposus, ◯ pulpous)

5. GERD – gastroesophageal (◯ reflex, ◯ reflux) disease

6. ILD – (◯ innerstitial, ◯ interstitial) lung disease

7. CHF – (◯ congestive, ◯ cardiac) heart failure

8. DJD – degenerative joint (◯ disorder, ◯ disease)

9. MS – (◯ megalo, ◯ multiple) sclerosis

10. CF – (◯ cerebral, ◯ cystic) fibrosis

Rooms – Lesson 1

Both physical locations in the hospital and individual hospital departments can have long names that can be slow to pronounce. In addition, both are referred to often in spoken and written medical reports. Following are some commonly used names with their abbreviations.

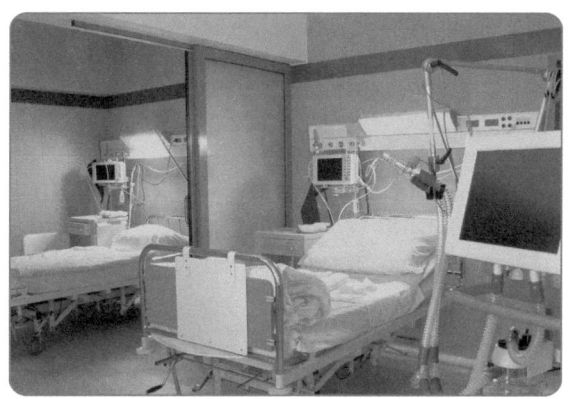

I. **ENTER ABBREVIATIONS.**
   Enter the abbreviation and what it stands for.

ER: emergency room
He was taken to the ER by paramedics.

   1. _____ (Abbreviation)

   2. _____

CCU: coronary care unit
Following CABG he was admitted to the CCU.

   3. _____ (Abbreviation)

   4. _____

ICU: intensive care unit
He was placed in the ICU upon admission.

   5. _____ (Abbreviation)

   6. _____

NICU: neonatal intensive care unit
The baby spent the first two weeks in the NICU.

   7. _____ (Abbreviation)

   8. _____

OR: operating room
He was taken to the OR for revision of TKA.

   9. _____ (Abbreviation)

   10. _____

PICU: pediatric intensive care unit
She spent two days in the PICU.

   11. _____ (Abbreviation)

   12. _____

SICU: surgical intensive care unit
There was no room in the SICU.

   13. _____ (Abbreviation)

   14. _____

II. FILL IN THE BLANK.
Expand the following abbreviations. For any abbreviation that has more than one expansion, just choose one that is appropriate for this lesson.

1. ICU _____   2. ER _____

3. OR _____   4. PICU _____

5. NICU _____   6. CCU _____

7. SICU _____

Departments – Lesson 2

I. ENTER ABBREVIATIONS.
Enter the abbreviation and what it stands for.

ENT: ears, nose, and throat
After consultation with ENT, a T&A was planned.

   1. _____ (Abbreviation)

   2. _____

GE: gastroenterology (not to be confused with gastroesophageal)
The GE service was consulted.

   3. _____ (Abbreviation)

   4. _____

The gastroenterology service is quite frequently referred to in dictation as the GI service. GI really stands for gastrointestinal; however, you will hear GI dictated far more than GE.

GYN: gynecology
She was being seen by Gynecology for her PID.

   5. _____ (Abbreviation)

   6. _____

OB: obstetrics
She will be followed up by her OB doctor.

   7. _____ (Abbreviation)

   8. _____

OT: occupational therapy
OT was called in for ADLs.

9. _____ (Abbreviation)

10. _____

PT: physical therapy
PT will instruct her on home exercises.

11. _____ (Abbreviation)

12. _____

II. FILL IN THE BLANK.
Expand the following abbreviations. For any abbreviation that has more than one expansion, just choose one that is appropriate for this lesson.

1. GYN_____   2. OB_____

3. ENT_____   4. GE_____

5. PT_____   6. OT_____

Weights and Measurements – Lesson 1

Precise measurements are a requirement in medicine for the simple reason that the wrong calculations can adversely affect patient care, whether a dosage measurement or a diagnostic lab study result. To that end, it is important to understand weight and measurement abbreviations. While the following lessons do not cover all units of weight and measurement abbreviations, they cover a healthy number of weight and measurement abbreviations used frequently in medical transcription.

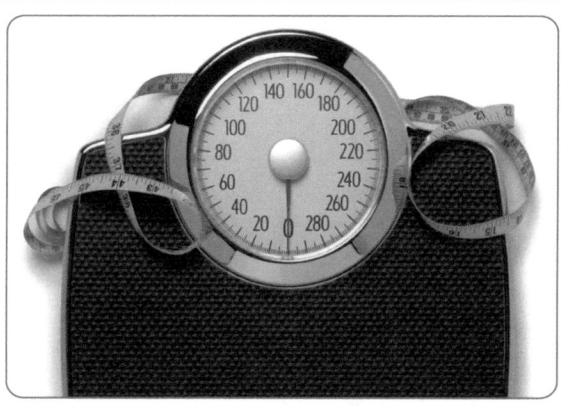

I. ENTER ABBREVIATIONS.
Enter the abbreviation and what it stands for.

cc: cubic centimeter
The dosage per patient is 0.50 cc into the anterior chamber.

1. _____ (Abbreviation)

2. _____

The abbreviation cc is on the ISMP List of Dangerous Abbreviations and some clients will prefer mL to be used in its place.

cGy: centigray
Radiation treatment at a dose of 500 cGy helps prevent clinically significant heterotopic ossification after total hip arthroplasty.

3. _____ (Abbreviation)

4. _____

dB: decibel
Noise levels of 85 dB and above are considered potentially damaging over time.

5. _____ (Abbreviation)

6. _____

cm: centimeter
A tagging suture was placed 5 cm above the greater trochanter.

7. _____ (Abbreviation)

8. _____

dL: deciliter
If the blood lead level of a child is greater than 10 mcg per dL, it may be considered abnormal.

9. _____ (Abbreviation)

10. _____

II. **FILL IN THE BLANK.**
   Some spaces may require more than one word. Be sure to provide the complete answer. For any question that may have more than one appropriate answer, just choose one.

1. A _____ is a unit used to express relative difference in power or intensity, usually between two acoustic or electric signals, equal to ten times the common logarithm of the ratio of the two levels.

2. A cubic _____ is a unit of volume equal to one thousandth of a liter, or to one milliliter.

3. A one-_____ dose of radiation is the equivalent of one rad.

4. One _____ is the equivalent of one tenth of a liter.

5. One _____ is the equivalent of one hundredth of a meter.

III. **FILL IN THE BLANK.**
   Expand the following abbreviations. For any abbreviation that has more than one expansion, just choose one that is appropriate for this lesson.

1. dB_____   2. cc_____

3. cGy_____   4. dL_____

5. cm_____

Weights and Measurements – Lesson 2

I. **ENTER ABBREVIATIONS.**
   Enter the abbreviation and what it stands for.

g or gm: gram
The patient was started on ampicillin 2 g and will receive this every 6 hours.

1. _____ (Abbreviation)

2. _____

While g and gm are appropriate abbreviations for gram, g is generally preferred.

Hz: hertz
Frequencies in Hz are usually written using the symbol f.

3. _____ (Abbreviation)

4. _____

L: liter
Due to her dehydrated state, the patient was given 1 L of fluids.

5. _____ (Abbreviation)

6. _____

mCi: millicurie
Patients participating in the trial received a radioactive dose of 40 mCi per week.

7. _____ (Abbreviation)

8. _____

mEq: milliequivalent
He was on diuretics, so he was additionally given potassium chloride 40 mEq per day.

9. _____ (Abbreviation)

10. _____

II. FILL IN THE BLANK.
Some spaces may require more than one word. Be sure to provide the complete answer. For any question that may have more than one appropriate answer, just choose one.

1. One _____ equals one thousandth of a kilogram.

2. The term _____ is a unit of frequency equal to 1 cycle per second.

3. A _____ is the metric equivalent of 0.264 gallons.

4. One _____ is a unit of radioactivity equal to one thousandth of a curie.

5. One _____ is equal to one thousandth of a compound's or an element's equivalent weight.

III. FILL IN THE BLANK.
Expand the following abbreviations. For any abbreviation that has more than one expansion, just choose one that is appropriate for this lesson.

1. L_____   2. mEq_____

3. Hz_____   4. g_____

5. mCi_____

Weights and Measurements – Lesson 3

I. ENTER ABBREVIATIONS.
Enter the abbreviation and what it stands for.

mg: milligram
Benadryl 50 mg was given to the patient at bedtime.

1. _____ (Abbreviation)

2. _____

mGy: milligray
The patient received a normal dose of 21.39 mGy during the CT scan.

3. _____ (Abbreviation)

4. _____

MHz: megahertz
Typical diagnostic sonographic scanners operate in the frequency range of 2 to 18 MHz.

5. _____ (Abbreviation)

6. _____

58

mL: milliliter
The doctor signed orders to administer normal saline at 83 mL per hour.

    7. _____ (Abbreviation)

    8. _____

mm: millimeter
A 2.5-mm incision was made to accommodate intraocular lens insertion.

    9. _____ (Abbreviation)

   10. _____

II. FILL IN THE BLANK.
Some spaces may require more than one word. Be sure to provide the complete answer. For any question that may have more than one appropriate answer, just choose one.

1. One _____ is equal to one thousandth of a gram.

2. One _____ is a unit of absorbed radiation equal to 0.001 gray.

3. The term _____ describes a unit of frequency equal to 1 million cycles per second.

4. A metric unit of measurement equal to one thousandth of a liter is called a _____.

5. A metric unit of length equal to one thousandth of a meter is called _____.

III. EXPAND THE FOLLOWING ABBREVIATIONS.
Expand the following abbreviations. For any abbreviation that has more than one expansion, just choose one that is appropriate for this lesson.

1. mL _____   2. mm _____

3. mGy _____   4. mg _____

5. MHz _____

Weights and Measurements – Lesson 4

I. ENTER ABBREVIATIONS.
Enter the abbreviation and what it stands for.

mmHg: millimeters of mercury
The patient's blood pressure was recorded as 135/65 mmHg.

    1. _____ (Abbreviation)

    2. _____

mmol: millimole
The low-dose solution contained 0.233 mmol of retinol.

    3. _____ (Abbreviation)

    4. _____

msec or ms: millisecond
The QT interval is measured by msec in an echocardiogram.

    5. _____ (Abbreviation)

    6. _____

m/sec: meters per second
The patient was able to achieve functional walking speeds averaging 1.1 m/sec.

    7. _____ (Abbreviation)

    8. _____

m/sec^2: meters per second squared
The aortic regurgitation tracing and profile revealed a slope of 4.7 m/sec^2.

    9. _____ (Abbreviation)

  10. _____

The 2 in m/sec^2 is normally typed as superscript; however, some platforms do not accommodate this, so it may be a style issue with regard to your particular employer.

nm: nanometer
The human eye normally has a peak spectral response of 550 nm.

  11. _____ (Abbreviation)

  12. _____

oz: ounce
The initial prescription of progesterone cream listed on the chart was 2 oz per day.

  13. _____ (Abbreviation)

  14. _____

II. FILL IN THE BLANK.
Some spaces may require more than one word. Be sure to provide the complete answer. For any question that may have more than one appropriate answer, just choose one.

    1. The abbreviation millimeters of _____ is used to reference blood pressure levels.

    2. One _____ is equal to one thousandth of a mole.

    3. One _____ is equal to one thousandth of a second.

4. The term m/sec refers to the distance measurement _____ per

    5. _____ .

6. The term m/sec^2 refers to distance measurement of _____ per second

    7. _____ .

8. The measurement of one billionth of a meter is referred to as a _____ .

9. An _____ is a unit of apothecary weight equal to 480 grains.

III. **FILL IN THE BLANK.**
Expand the following abbreviations. For any abbreviation that has more than one expansion, just choose one that is appropriate for this lesson.

1. nm _____   2. m/sec _____

3. oz _____   4. mmol _____

5. mmHg _____   6. msec _____

7. m/sec^2 _____

Review: Weights and Measurements

I. **MATCHING.**
Match the term to the correct abbreviation.

1. ____ hertz   A. mL

2. ____ centigray   B. mEq

                         C. mCi

3. ____ milliequivalent   D. Hz

4. ____ milliliter   E. g

5. ____ nanometer   F. mg

                         G. oz

6. ____ ounce   H. L

7. ____ liter   I. cGy

8. ____ milligram   J. nm

9. ____ gram

10. ____ millicurie

II. FILL IN THE BLANK.
Expand the following abbreviations. For any abbreviation that has more than one expansion, just choose one that is appropriate for this lesson.

1. dL_____

2. MHz_____

3. cc_____

4. msec_____

5. mm_____

6. m/sec_____

7. mGy_____

8. cm_____

9. mmol_____

10. Hz_____

11. dB_____

12. mmHg_____

13. m/sec^2_____

Abbreviations by Specialty

The following lessons include abbreviations categorized by specialty. Again, this is done in an effort to help you not only associate the letters themselves with their respective meanings, but also with their appropriate context. The specialties to be covered include:
- Cardiology
- OB/GYN
- Orthopedics
- Radiology
- Surgery

All specialties have related abbreviations and therefore this is obviously not an exhaustive list of specialty-related abbreviations. These are, however, some of the most common specialty-related abbreviations you will be exposed to. Pay attention to the classification into which each abbreviation fits, as it will assist you in learning these abbreviations thoroughly and what they stand for.

Cardiology – Lesson 1

The heart is one of the most complex structures of the body. Cardiology refers to the study of the heart and treatment of heart disease. Cardiac catheterizations and heart surgeries deal with intricate veins and arteries, several of which are abbreviated. Following are abbreviations of heart problems, procedures, and structures.

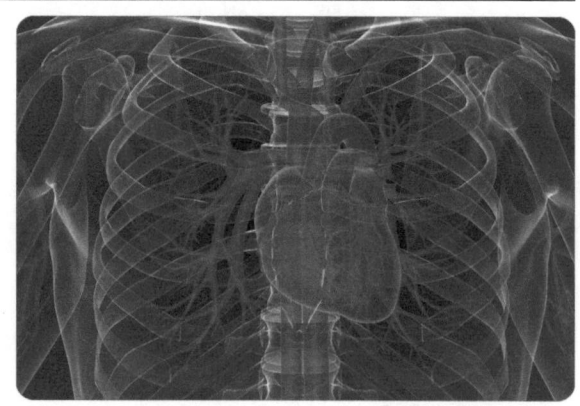

I. ENTER ABBREVIATIONS.
Enter the abbreviation and what it stands for.

A-fib: atrial fibrillation
He went into A-fib.

    1. _____ (Abbreviation)

    2. _____

ASCAD: arteriosclerotic coronary artery disease (atherosclerotic coronary artery disease)
His past medical history is significant for ASCAD.

    3. _____ (Abbreviation)

    4. _____

ACLS: advanced cardiac life support
The patient was given ACLS.

    5. _____ (Abbreviation)

    6. _____

ASCVD: arteriosclerotic cardiovascular disease (atherosclerotic cardiovascular disease)
Cardiac catheterization revealed advanced ASCVD.

    7. _____ (Abbreviation)

    8. _____

ASHD: arteriosclerotic heart disease (atherosclerotic heart disease)
On family history, it was discovered that both the patient's parents died of ASHD.

    9. _____ (Abbreviation)

    10. _____

AV: atrioventricular
AV nodal ablation was performed to correct chronic atrial fibrillation.

    11. _____ (Abbreviation)

    12. _____

II. FILL IN THE BLANK.
Some spaces may require more than one word. Be sure to provide the complete answer. For any question that may have more than one appropriate answer, just choose one.

    1. She was in atrial _____ on admission.

    2. Her _____ coronary artery disease required CABG.

    3. She was taken off advanced _____ life support.

4. _____ heart disease is exacerbated by smoking.

5. There was an atrio _____ groove.

6. The patient was 95 years old and had no evidence of atherosclerotic cardio _____ disease.

III. **FILL IN THE BLANK.**
Expand the following abbreviations. For any abbreviation that has more than one expansion, just choose one that is appropriate for this lesson.

1. ASCAD _____   2. ASCVD _____

3. AV _____   4. A-fib _____

5. ASHD _____   6. ACLS _____

Cardiology – Lesson 2

I. **ENTER ABBREVIATIONS.**
Enter the abbreviation and what it stands for.

CABG: coronary artery bypass grafting
He underwent CABG for severe three-vessel disease.

1. _____ (Abbreviation)

2. _____

This abbreviation is often pronounced "cabbage," although it can be C-A-B-G.

ECG/EKG: electrocardiogram (electrocardiography)
His EKG showed an ST depression.

3. _____ (Abbreviation)

4. _____

EF: ejection fraction
Her ejection fraction was 23%.

5. _____ (Abbreviation)

6. _____

fem-fem: femoral-femoral
The patient had coronary artery bypass graft with fem-fem anastomosis.

  7. _____ (Abbreviation)

  8. _____

fem-pop: femoral-popliteal
A femoral-popliteal bypass was performed due to blockage of the patient's femoral artery.

  9. _____ (Abbreviation)

  10. _____

II. **FILL IN THE BLANK.**
   Some spaces may require more than one word. Be sure to provide the complete answer. For any question that may have more than one appropriate answer, just choose one.

  1. "We then performed the _____ -pop anastomosis."

  2. Coronary _____ bypass [3.]_____ times four was planned.

  4. There was an _____ fraction of 26%.

  5. An _____ gram was performed and was entirely normal.

  6. Tissue for the fem-_____ portion of the surgery was taken from the right leg.

III. **FILL IN THE BLANK.**
   Expand the following abbreviations. For any abbreviation that has more than one expansion, just choose one that is appropriate for this lesson.

  1. EF _____   2. CABG _____

  3. fem-fem _____   4. fem-pop _____

  5. ECG _____ .

Cardiology – Lesson 3

I. **ENTER ABBREVIATIONS.**
   Enter the abbreviation and what it stands for.

  IVC: inferior vena cava
  The IVC was spared.

  1. _____ (Abbreviation)

  2. _____

LAD: left anterior descending (artery)
The LAD was free of disease.

    3. _____ (Abbreviation)

    4. _____

LAO: left anterior oblique
Films were taken in the LAO projection.

    5. _____ (Abbreviation)

    6. _____

LCA: left coronary artery (left circumflex artery)
The LCA had a 30% plaque.

    7. _____ (Abbreviation)

    8. _____

LIMA: left internal mammary artery
Her LIMA was unaffected by disease.

    9. _____ (Abbreviation)

    10. _____

This is often pronounced "LIMA," with an ee sound for the I.

II. FILL IN THE BLANK.
Some spaces may require more than one word. Be sure to provide the complete answer. For any question that may have more than one appropriate answer, just choose one.

    1. The left _____ descending artery was normal.

    2. The _____ internal 3._____ artery was free of disease.

    4. The right _____ vena 5._____ was normal.

    6. The left anterior _____ position was utilized.

    7. The left _____ artery is occluded.

III. FILL IN THE BLANK.
Expand the following abbreviations. For any abbreviation that has more than one expansion, just choose one that is appropriate for this lesson.

1. LCA _____   2. LIMA _____

3. IVC _____   4. LAO _____

5. LAD _____

Cardiology – Lesson 4

I. ENTER ABBREVIATIONS.
Enter the abbreviation and what it stands for.

LV: left ventricle (ventricular)
Normal LV function.

1. _____ (Abbreviation)

2. _____

MI: myocardial infarction
She has a history of MI two years ago.

3. _____ (Abbreviation)

4. _____

OMB: obtuse marginal branch
Her OMB was totally occluded.

5. _____ (Abbreviation)

6. _____

PDA: patent ductus arteriosus (posterior descending artery)
The infant had a PDA.
Evidence of ASCAD was found in the PDA.

7. _____ (Abbreviation)

8. _____

9. _____

PE: pulmonary embolism (embolus)
Ventilation/perfusion scan indicated a possible PE.

10. _____ (Abbreviation)

11. _____

PTCA: percutaneous transluminal coronary angioplasty
She presents for cardiac catheterization and probable PTCA.

12. _____ (Abbreviation)

13. _____

PVC: premature ventricular contraction
She had persistent PVCs.

14. _____ (Abbreviation)

15. _____

PVD: peripheral vascular disease
Coolness of his extremities was consistent with PVD.

16. _____ (Abbreviation)

17. _____

II. FILL IN THE BLANK.
Some spaces may require more than one word. Be sure to provide the complete answer. For any question that may have more than one appropriate answer, just choose one.

1. She has a history of premature _____.

2. _____ infarction was ruled out.

3. She had an occluded _____ marginal branch.

4. _____ coronary 5._____ was attempted.

6. She has normal left _____ function.

7. Given his history, pulmonary _____ was part of the differential diagnosis.

8. The infant was diagnosed with _____ arteriosus.

9. The PTCA showed 80% occlusion of the posterior _____ artery.

10. _____ vascular disease is the cause of deep venous thrombosis.

III. FILL IN THE BLANK.
Expand the following abbreviations. For any abbreviation that has more than one expansion, just choose one that is appropriate for this lesson.

1. OMB _____   2. LV _____

3. PVC _____   4. MI _____

5. PTCA _____   6. PDA _____

7. PE _____   8. PVD _____

Cardiology – Lesson 5

I. **ENTER ABBREVIATIONS.**
   Enter the abbreviation and what it stands for.

RAD: right anterior descending (artery)
She had a normal RAD.

   1. _____ (Abbreviation)

   2. _____

RAO: right anterior oblique
Films were taken in RAO and LAO projections.

   3. _____ (Abbreviation)

   4. _____

RCA: right coronary artery
She had a totally occluded RCA.

   5. _____ (Abbreviation)

   6. _____

Occasionally, this can also be right circumflex artery.

SMA: superior mesenteric artery
His SMA was damaged in the accident.

   7. _____ (Abbreviation)

   8. _____

SMA also has reference to a panel of laboratory tests.

SVC: superior vena cava
His SVC was visualized.

   9. _____ (Abbreviation)

   10. _____

V-tach: ventricular tachycardia
The patient went into acute V-tach.

   11. _____ (Abbreviation)

   12. _____

II. FILL IN THE BLANK.
Some spaces may require more than one word. Be sure to provide the complete answer. For any question that may have more than one appropriate answer, just choose one.

1. The right _____ oblique position was used.

2. The right _____ artery was damaged.

3. The patient went into _____ tachycardia.

4. The superior _____ was within normal limits.

5. Right anterior _____ artery was totally occluded.

6. Superior _____ artery is found in the abdomen.

III. FILL IN THE BLANK.
Expand the following abbreviations. For any abbreviation that has more than one expansion, just choose one that is appropriate for this lesson.

1. V-tach _____

2. SVC _____

3. RAD _____

4. RCA _____

5. RAO _____

6. SMA _____

Review: Cardiology

I. FILL IN THE BLANK.
Using the word/word parts in the box, enter the appropriate term in the space provided.

1. premature _____ contractions

2. ventricular _____

3. right _____ oblique

4. inferior _____ cava

5. patent ductus _____

6. left anterior _____

7. peripheral _____ disease

8. left internal _____ artery

9. _____ vena cava

10. _____ infarction

anterior
arteriosus
descending
mammary
myocardial
superior
tachycardia
vascular
vena
ventricular

II. MATCHING.
Match the word or word part to the abbreviation expansion.

1. ____ V-tach – _____ tachycardia

2. ____ CABG – coronary artery bypass _____

3. ____ PTCA – percutaneous _____ coronary angioplasty

4. ____ EF – _____ fraction

5. ____ LCA – left _____ artery

6. ____ PE – pulmonary _____

7. ____ SMA – superior _____ artery

8. ____ RAO – right anterior _____

9. ____ ASHD – _____ heart disease

10. ____ LCA – _____ coronary artery

A. ejection
B. oblique
C. ventricular
D. grafting
E. embolism
F. mesenteric
G. left
H. transluminal
I. atherosclerotic
J. circumflex

III. MULTIPLE CHOICE.
Choose the best answer.

1. LV
   - ○ leftover ventricle
   - ○ lead ventricle
   - ○ left ventricle
   - ○ left ventrical

2. OMB
   - ○ obtuse marginal branch
   - ○ outer marginal branch
   - ○ obtuse main branch
   - ○ outer margin brachial

3. PDA
   - ○ patient ductus arteriosus
   - ○ patent ductis artiosis
   - ○ patent ductus arteriosis
   - ○ patent ductus arteriosus

4. PVD
   - ○ premature ventricular disease
   - ○ peripheral vascular disease
   - ○ peripheral ventricular disease
   - ○ premature vascular disease

5. fem-pop
   - ○ femoral-popliteal
   - ○ femoral-poplitial
   - ○ female-poplitial
   - ○ femoral-popaliteal

6. ASCAD
   - ○ arteriosclerotic cardiac anginal disease
   - ○ artriosclerotic coronary artery disease
   - ○ arteriosclerotic coronary artery disease
   - ○ arteriosclerotic cardiovascular artery disease

7. A-fib
   ○ anterior fibula
   ○ anterior fibrillation
   ○ atrial fibrilation
   ○ atrial fibrillation

8. ACLS
   ○ advanced coronary living support
   ○ advanced cardiac life support
   ○ atherosclerotic coronary life support
   ○ arteriosclerotic cardiovascular life support

9. IVC
   ○ inferior venous cardiography
   ○ inferior venous cava
   ○ inferior vena cava
   ○ inner vena cava

10. MI
    ○ myocardial infarction
    ○ mycardial infarction
    ○ myocardial infraction
    ○ myocardile infarction

Fetal Measurements – Lesson 1

Obstetrics and Gynecology is a field that frequently uses abbreviations. They are used especially for terms dealing with pregnancy, as this is obviously a common condition. Following are abbreviated terms that you will use often in all kinds of OB/GYN reports, as well as histories for female patients. These abbreviations are broken down into related groups.

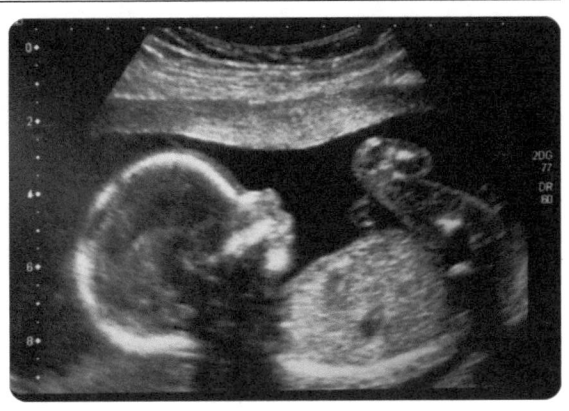

I. **ENTER ABBREVIATIONS.**
    Enter the abbreviation and what it stands for.

    AC: abdominal circumference
    1. _____ (Abbreviation)
    2. _____

BPD: biparietal diameter
   3. _____ (Abbreviation)
   4. _____

EFW: estimated fetal weight
   5. _____ (Abbreviation)
   6. _____

FL: femur length
   7. _____ (Abbreviation)
   8. _____

HC: head circumference
   9. _____ (Abbreviation)
   10. _____

MEASUREMENTS: BPD 8.3 cm for 32.1 weeks, HC 11.0 cm for 32.6 weeks, AC 14.2 cm for 33.1 weeks, and FL 4.5 cm for 32.8 weeks.

II. **FILL IN THE BLANK.**
Expand the following abbreviations. For any abbreviation that has more than one expansion, just choose one appropriate for this lesson.

1. BPD_____   2. FL_____

3. EFW_____   4. AC_____

5. HC_____

General History – Lesson 2

I. **ENTER ABBREVIATIONS.**
Enter the abbreviation and what it stands for.

AB: abortion or abortus
(can also be written "ab")
   1. _____ (Abbreviation)
   2. _____

G: gravida (# of pregnancies)
   3. _____ (Abbreviation)
   4. _____

P: para (# of living children)

    5. _____ (Abbreviation)

    6. _____

SAB: spontaneous abortion

    7. _____ (Abbreviation)

    8. _____

TAB: therapeutic abortion

    9. _____ (Abbreviation)

    10. _____

The patient is a G5, P3, AB2 (SAB 1, TAB 1).

II. FILL IN THE BLANK.
Expand the following abbreviations. For any abbreviation that has more than one expansion, just choose one appropriate for this lesson.

1. G _____   2. AB _____

3. SAB _____   4. P _____

5. TAB _____

Obstetrical Terms – Lesson 3

I. ENTER ABBREVIATIONS.
Enter the abbreviation and what it stands for.

C-section: cesarean section
The patient has a history of C-section times two in the past.

    1. _____ (Abbreviation)

    2. _____

CPD: cephalopelvic disproportion
C-section was performed secondary to CPD.

    3. _____ (Abbreviation)

    4. _____

EDC: estimated date of confinement
She has a gestational age of 26.4 weeks, giving her an EDC of 2-12-94.

    5. _____ (Abbreviation)

    6. _____

EGA: estimated gestational age
The patient has an EGA of 32.9 weeks.

   7. _____ (Abbreviation)

   8. _____

IUGR: intrauterine growth retardation
There is evidence of IUGR.

   9. _____ (Abbreviation)

   10. _____

II. **FILL IN THE BLANK.**
   Some spaces may require more than one word. Be sure to provide the complete answer.

   1. She underwent elective _____ section without complications.

   2. Ultrasound dates gave her an estimated date of _____ of 13 April 91.

   3. She should return for a followup ultrasound because of _____ growth
      4. _____.

   5. She underwent pelvimetry for possible _____ disproportion.

   6. She has an _____ gestational age of 22.4 weeks.

Obstetrical Terms – Lesson 4

I. **ENTER ABBREVIATIONS.**
   Enter the abbreviation and what it stands for.

   L&D: labor and delivery
   The patient was taken to L&D and delivered triplets.

   1. _____ (Abbreviation)

   2. _____

   LGA: large for gestational age
   The fetus shows an LGA growth curve.

   3. _____ (Abbreviation)

   4. _____

   LMP: last menstrual period
   Her LMP is 18 June, giving her an EDC of 28 March.

   5. _____ (Abbreviation)

   6. _____

MSAFP: maternal serum alpha fetoprotein
She is MSAFP negative.

    7. _____ (Abbreviation)

    8. _____

NSVD: normal spontaneous vaginal delivery
She was admitted and had an NSVD.

    9. _____ (Abbreviation)

   10. _____

ROM: rupture of membranes
She had spontaneous ROM before coming to the hospital.

   11. _____ (Abbreviation)

   12. _____

VBAC: vaginal birth after cesarean (Usually pronounced V-back)
The patient wished to attempt VBAC.

   13. _____ (Abbreviation)

   14. _____

II. FILL IN THE BLANK.
Some spaces may require more than one word. Be sure to provide the complete answer.

    1. Her last _____ period was in 1978.

    2. She had normal _____ vaginal delivery.

    3. She was a large for _____ age baby.

    4. Maternal serum _____ was normal.

    5. _____ after cesarean was attempted.

    6. She presented to the ER with _____ of membranes.

    7. She was in labor and _____ for 36 hours.

FILL IN THE BLANK.
Expand the following abbreviations. For any abbreviation that has more than one expansion, just choose one appropriate for this lesson.

1. LGA _____ 2. C-section _____

3. LMP _____ 4. CPD _____

5. MSAFP _____ 6. IUGR _____

7. EDC _____ 8. EGA _____

9. ROM _____ 10. NSVD _____

11. VBAC _____ 12. L&D _____

Gynecology Terms – Lesson 5

I. **ENTER ABBREVIATIONS.**
Enter the abbreviation and what it stands for.

BSO: bilateral salpingo-oophorectomy
She underwent TAH-BSO in 1974.

1. _____ (Abbreviation)

2. _____

D&C: dilatation and curettage (dilation and curettage)
She had a D&C as treatment for intermenstrual bleeding.

3. _____ (Abbreviation)

4. _____

PID: pelvic inflammatory disease
She was sent to the emergency room for possible PID.

5. _____ (Abbreviation)

6. _____

TAH: total abdominal hysterectomy (often TAH-BSO)
She had a TAH performed immediately following cesarean section.

7. _____ (Abbreviation)

8. _____

TVH: total vaginal hysterectomy
She presents for TVH.

9. _____ (Abbreviation)

10. _____

II. FILL IN THE BLANK.
Some spaces may require more than one word. Be sure to provide the complete answer.

1. She is having infertility problems secondary to a history of pelvic _____ disease.

2. Bilateral _____-oophorectomy was performed secondary to a cystic mass on the left ovary.

3. Total abdominal _____ was performed.

4. Total _____ hysterectomy was performed.

5. Dilatation and _____ was indicated for hypermenorrhea.

III. FILL IN THE BLANK.
Expand the following abbreviations. For any abbreviation that has more than one expansion, just choose one appropriate for this lesson.

1. TAH-BSO _____

2. TVH _____

3. D&C _____

4. PID _____

5. BSO _____

Review: OB/GYN

I. FILL IN THE BLANK.

Some spaces may require more than one word. Be sure to provide the complete answer. For any question that may have more than one appropriate answer, just choose one.

1. abdominal _____

2. cephalopelvic _____

3. pelvic _____ disease

4. spontaneous _____

5. _____ date of confinement

6. last menstrual _____

7. intrauterine _____ retardation

8. total abdominal _____

9. _____ length

10. bilateral salpingo-_____

abortion
circumference
disproportion
estimated
femur
growth
hysterectomy
inflammatory
oophorectomy
period

II. MULTIPLE CHOICE.

Choose the correct word or word part for the abbreviation expansion.

1. CPD – (◯craniopelvic, ◯ cephalopelvic) disproportion

2. TAB – (◯therapeutic, ◯ total) abortion

3. AC – (◯amniotic, ◯ abdominal) circumference

4. EDC – estimated date of (◯cesarean, ◯ confinement)

5. LGA – large for (◯gestational, ◯ genetic) age

6. VBAC – vaginal birth after (◯cesarean, ◯ confinement)

7. MSAFP – maternal serum (◯after, ◯ alpha) fetoprotein

8. FL – (◯femur, ◯ fetal) length

9. EFW – (◯exact,◯ estimated) fetal weight

10. HC – (◯head,◯ heart) circumference

III. MATCHING.
Match the word or word part to the abbreviation expansion.

1. ____ SAB – _____ abortion

2. ____ G – _____

3. ____ BPD – biparietal _____

4. ____ ROM – rupture of _____

5. ____ D&C – _____ and curettage

6. ____ P – _____

7. ____ TVH – total _____ hysterectomy

8. ____ PID – pelvic _____ disease

9. ____ L&D – labor and _____

10. ____ IUGR – _____ growth retardation

A. diameter
B. membrane
C. gravida
D. spontaneous
E. intrauterine
F. dilatation
G. delivery
H. vaginal
I. para
J. inflammatory

Orthopedics – Lesson 1

Orthopedics is a branch of medicine concerned with the skeletal system, its articulation, and its associated structures. The following exercises introduce abbreviations related to bones/joints and associated ligaments.

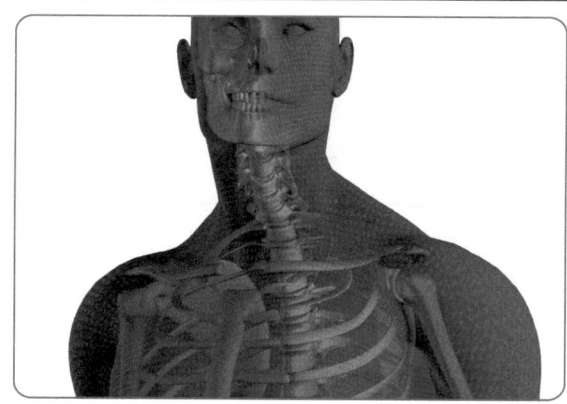

I. ENTER ABBREVIATIONS.
Enter the abbreviation and what it stands for.

AC: acromioclavicular
The AC joint is intact.

1. _____ (Abbreviation)

2. _____

ACL: anterior cruciate ligament
There is evidence of a torn ACL.

    3. _____ (Abbreviation)

    4. _____

AFO: ankle-foot orthosis (ankle-foot orthotic)
He required AFO for his malleolar deformity.

    5. _____ (Abbreviation)

    6. _____

C-spine: cervical spine
The C-spine was imaged.

    7. _____ (Abbreviation)

    8. _____

CMC: carpometacarpal (joint)
The CMC is normal.

    9. _____ (Abbreviation)

    10. _____

DDD: degenerative disc disease
Spinal x-rays revealed DDD.

    11. _____ (Abbreviation)

    12. _____

DIP: distal interphalangeal (joint)
There is no DIP separation.

    13. _____ (Abbreviation)

    14. _____

II. **FILL IN THE BLANK.**
    Some spaces may require more than one word. Be sure to provide the complete answer. For any question that may have more than one appropriate answer, just choose one.

    1. The acromio _____ joint is separated.

    2. There is no anterior _____ ligament instability.

    3. The _____ spine is within normal limits.

    4. The _____ metacarpal is normal.

    5. The distal _____ joint is intact.

6. His ankle-foot _____ helped to alleviate the problem.

7. His _____ disc disease caused him great pain.

III. **FILL IN THE BLANK.**
   Expand the following abbreviations. For any abbreviation that has more than one expansion, just choose one that is appropriate for this lesson.

1. DIP _____   2. AC _____

3. CMC _____   4. C-spine _____

5. ACL _____   6. AFO _____

7. DDD _____

Orthopedics – Lesson 2

I. **ENTER ABBREVIATIONS.**
   Enter the abbreviation and what it stands for.

IP: interphalangeal
The IP joint is intact.

1. _____ (Abbreviation)

2. _____

IT: iliotibial
The iliotibial band is visualized and is within normal limits.

3. _____ (Abbreviation)

4. _____

L-spine: lumbar spine
A lumbar spine film was done.

5. _____ (Abbreviation)

6. _____

LS: lumbosacral (spine)
The lumbosacral spine film is normal.

7. _____ (Abbreviation)

8. _____

MCL: medial collateral ligament
He injured his MCL playing football.

    9. _____ (Abbreviation)

    10. _____

MCP: metacarpophalangeal (joint)
The MCP joint is unremarkable.

    11. _____ (Abbreviation)

    12. _____

II. FILL IN THE BLANK.
Some spaces may require more than one word. Be sure to provide the complete answer. For any question that may have more than one appropriate answer, just choose one.

    1. The _____ band is intact.

    2. The _____ phalangeal joint is unremarkable.

    3. Lumbo _____ spine is within normal limits.

    4. The right inter _____ joint was visualized.

    5. There is slight straightening of the _____ spine.

    6. Medial _____ ligament was assessed by arthroscopy.

III. FILL IN THE BLANK.
Expand the following abbreviations. For any abbreviation that has more than one expansion, just choose one that is appropriate for this lesson.

    1. MCP _____   2. L-spine _____

    3. IP _____   4. LS _____

    5. IT _____   6. MCL _____

Orthopedics – Lesson 3

I. **ENTER ABBREVIATIONS.**
   Enter the abbreviation and what it stands for.

MTP: metatarsophalangeal (joint)
The MTP joint is normal.

   1. _____ (Abbreviation)

   2. _____

PCL: posterior cruciate ligament
No laxity of the PCL.

   3. _____ (Abbreviation)

   4. _____

PIP: proximal interphalangeal
The PIP joint is unremarkable.

   5. _____ (Abbreviation)

   6. _____

SI: sacroiliac (joint)
The SI joints were scanned and were within normal limits.

   7. _____ (Abbreviation)

   8. _____

T-spine: thoracic spine
The thoracic spine was imaged from T1–T12.

   9. _____ (Abbreviation)

   10. _____

tib-fib: tibial-fibular or tibiofibular
X-ray showed a right tib-fib fracture.

   11. _____ (Abbreviation)

   12. _____

The abbreviation tib-fib is nearly always used as an adjective. Occasionally, however, it is used as a noun (tibia-fibula).

TMJ: temporomandibular joint
The TMJ moved normally.

   13. _____ (Abbreviation)

   14. _____

II. FILL IN THE BLANK.
Some spaces may require more than one word. Be sure to provide the complete answer. For any question that may have more than one appropriate answer, just choose one.

1. The _____ cruciate ligament is intact.

2. The _____ mandibular joint is imaged.

3. _____ iliac joints appear intact.

4. AP and lateral views of the _____ spine were obtained.

5. The _____ interphalangeal joint appears intact.

6. On views of the right foot, the _____ phalangeal joint was noted to be separated.

7. The tibial-_____ fracture was casted.

III. FILL IN THE BLANK.
Expand the following abbreviations. For any abbreviation that has more than one expansion, just choose one that is appropriate for this lesson.

1. MTP _____

2. SI _____

3. T-spine _____

4. TMJ _____

5. PCL _____

6. PIP _____

7. tib-fib _____

Review: Orthopedics

I. FILL IN THE BLANK.
Using the word/word parts in the box, enter the appropriate term in the space provided.

1. tibial-_____

2. acromio _____

3. degenerative _____ disease

4. lumbo _____

5. _____ carpal

6. ilio _____

7. medial _____ ligament

8. ankle-foot _____

9. posterior _____ ligament

10. distal _____

carpometa
clavicular
collateral
cruciate
disc
fibular
interphalangeal
orthosis
sacral
tibial

II. MATCHING.
Match the word or word part for the appropriate abbreviation expansion. A term may be used more than once.

1. ____ SI – _____ iliac

2. ____ MCP – metacarpo _____

3. ____ TMJ – _____ joint

4. ____ L-spine – _____ spine

5. ____ IP – inter _____

6. ____ ACL – anterior _____

7. ____ PIP – proximal _____

8. ____ C-spine – _____ spine

9. ____ MTP – metatarso _____

10. ____ T-spine – _____ spine

A. temporomandibular
B. cruciate ligament
C. phalangeal
D. sacro
E. meta
F. cervical
G. lumbar
H. interphalangeal
I. thoracic

III. MULTIPLE CHOICE.
Choose the best answer.

1. AFO

    ○ ankle for orthosis
    ○ another foot orthopedic
    ○ ankle-foot orthosis
    ○ ankle-foot orthopedic

2. DIP

    ○ dorsal interphalangeal
    ○ distal interphalangeal
    ○ distal innerphalangeal
    ○ dorsum innerspace proximal

3. LS

    ○ lumbosacral
    ○ lumbasacrol
    ○ lumbasacral
    ○ lumbosacrol

4. AC

    ○ acromoclavicular
    ○ aceromyoclavicular
    ○ acromioclavicular
    ○ acromyoclaviculer

5. DDD

    ○ disc disease degeneration
    ○ degenerating disease of the discs
    ○ disco degeneration disease
    ○ degenerative disc disease

6. PCL

    ○ posterior cruciate ligament
    ○ proximal cruciate ligament
    ○ proximal clavicular ligament
    ○ posterior clavicular ligament

7. IT
   - ○ interotibial
   - ○ innertibial
   - ○ iliotibial
   - ○ ileotibial

8. TMJ
   - ○ temporamandible joint
   - ○ temporomandicular joint
   - ○ temporomandibular joint
   - ○ temperomandibular joint

9. PIP
   - ○ posterior innerphalangeal
   - ○ posterior interphalangeal
   - ○ proximal innerphalangeal
   - ○ proximal interphalangeal

10. CMC
   - ○ carpometacruciate
   - ○ carpometacarpal
   - ○ claviculometacarpal
   - ○ claviculometaclavicular

Radiology – Lesson 1

When you think of an x-ray, you generally think of a picture of a specific bone or the chest. The field of radiology, however, includes several other types of scans and procedures. Following are some of the most frequently used radiology abbreviations.

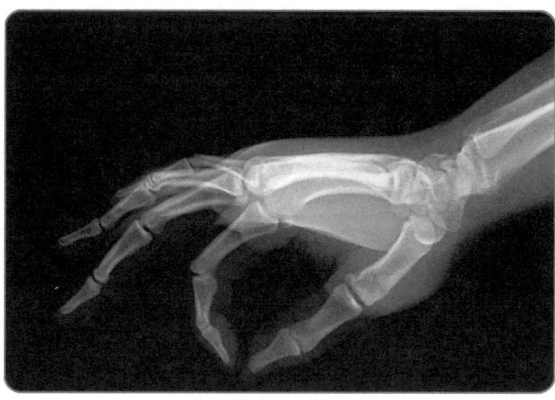

I. ENTER ABBREVIATIONS.
Enter the abbreviation and what it stands for.

AP/PA: anteroposterior/posteroanterior
PA chest was performed.

    1. _____ (Abbreviation)

    2. _____

BE: barium enema
After GI consult, BE was performed.

    3. _____ (Abbreviation)

    4. _____

CT: computed tomography
A CT scan of the abdomen and pelvis was carried out.

    5. _____ (Abbreviation)

    6. _____

EEG: electroencephalogram
As part of her sleep workup an EEG was performed.

    7. _____ (Abbreviation)

    8. _____

ERCP: endoscopic retrograde cholangiopancreatography
ERCP was performed.

    9. _____ (Abbreviation)

    10. _____

GI: gastrointestinal
An upper GI with small bowel follow-through was performed.

    11. _____ (Abbreviation)

    12. _____

Upper GI is the common term for an examination of that area.

II. FILL IN THE BLANK.
Some spaces may require more than one word. Be sure to provide the complete answer. For any question that may have more than one appropriate answer, just choose one.

    1. The chest was photographed in the antero_____ dimension.

    2. An electro _____ was performed.

3. An upper _____ exam was normal.

4. _____ tomography images were taken of the brain.

5. An endoscopic retrograde _____ was ordered.

6. _____ enema was within normal limits.

III. FILL IN THE BLANK.
Expand the following abbreviations. For any abbreviation that has more than one expansion, just choose one that is appropriate for this lesson.

1. ERCP_____   2. BE _____

3. CT _____   4. EEG _____

5. GI _____   6. AP/PA _____

Radiology – Lesson 2

I. ENTER ABBREVIATIONS.
Enter the abbreviation and what it stands for.

HIDA: hydroxyiminodiacetic acid
A HIDA scan was done.

1. _____ (Abbreviation)

2. _____

This is pronounced "hida" (with a long i sound as in "find"). The individual letters are not dictated out.

IVP: intravenous pyelogram
An IVP was entirely within normal limits.

3. _____ (Abbreviation)

4. _____

KUB: kidneys, ureters, bladder (abdominal x-ray)
KUB was performed.

5. _____ (Abbreviation)

6. _____

MRI: magnetic resonance imaging
An MRI of the chest, abdomen, and pelvis was carried out.

7. _____ (Abbreviation)

8. _____

MUGA: multiple gated acquisition
On MUGA images there were no abnormalities.

9. _____ (Abbreviation)

10. _____

This is pronounced "mugga," and it is nearly always dictated that way.

OCG: oral cholecystogram
She had an OCG which was negative.

11. _____ (Abbreviation)

12. _____

VCUG: voiding cystourethrogram
VCUG showed no abnormalities.

13. _____ (Abbreviation)

14. _____

II. FILL IN THE BLANK.
Some spaces may require more than one word. Be sure to provide the complete answer. For any question that may have more than one appropriate answer, just choose one.

1. A _____ acid scan was performed.

2. _____ pyelogram was ordered.

3. The doctor ordered a _____, ureters, and 4._____ x-ray.

5. Multiple _____ scan was normal.

6. _____ resonance imaging of the brain was performed.

7. An oral _____ was done.

8. Voiding _____ was normal.

III. **FILL IN THE BLANK.**
Expand the following abbreviations. For any abbreviation that has more than one expansion, just choose one that is appropriate for this lesson.

1. MUGA_____   2. IVP_____

3. MRI_____   4. HIDA_____

5. KUB_____   6. VCUG_____

7. OCG_____

Review: Radiology

I. **FILL IN THE BLANK.**
Using the word/word parts in the box, enter the appropriate term in the space provided.

1. antero _____

2. _____ cholecystogram

3. multiple _____

4. endoscopic _____

5. upper _____

6. _____encephalogram

7. kidneys, _____, bladder

8. _____ tomography

9. _____ cystourethrogram

10. _____ resonance 11._____

12. hydroxy _____ acid

13. intravenous _____

14. barium _____

computed
electro
enema
gastrointestinal
gated acquisition
imaging
iminodiacetic
magnetic
oral
posterior
pyelogram
retrograde cholangio-pancreatography
ureters
voiding

II. MULTIPLE CHOICE.
Choose the best answer.

1. EEG
   - ◯ electroechocardiogram
   - ◯ electroencephalography
   - ◯ electroencephalogram
   - ◯ echoenceophalogram

2. BE
   - ◯ barioenema
   - ◯ barium enema
   - ◯ barium encephalogram
   - ◯ bladder electrography

3. PA
   - ◯ proximal anterior
   - ◯ proximoanteral
   - ◯ posterioranterior
   - ◯ posteroanterior

4. IVP
   - ◯ intestinopyelogram
   - ◯ intraventricular pancreatography
   - ◯ intraventricular pyelogram
   - ◯ intravenous pyelogram

5. MRI
   - ◯ magnetic resonance imaging
   - ◯ magnetic rhythm incephalogram
   - ◯ macrorythm imaging
   - ◯ magneticrecognizanceimagery

6. GI
   - ◯ genitointestinal
   - ◯ genitointravenous
   - ◯ gastrointestinal
   - ◯ gastrointestinle

7. CT

  ○ computer tomography

  ○ computer topography

  ○ computed topography

  ○ computed tomography

8. KUB

  ○ kidneys under bladder

  ○ kidneys, urethra, bladder

  ○ kidneys, ureters, bladder

  ○ kidneys, uvula, bladder

9. OCG

  ○ oral cystogram

  ○ oral cholangiopancreatography

  ○ oral computed gramography

  ○ oral cholecystogram

10. MUGA

  ○ magnetic upper gaited acquisition

  ○ multiple gaited acquisition

  ○ multiple gastric acquisition

  ○ multiple gated acquisition

Surgery – Lesson 1

I. **ENTER ABBREVIATIONS.**
Enter the abbreviation and what it stands for.

AKA: above-knee amputation
Examination of the lower extremities revealed a right AKA.

  1. _____ (Abbreviation)

  2. _____

BKA: below-knee amputation
History of BKA in 1969.

  3. _____ (Abbreviation)

  4. _____

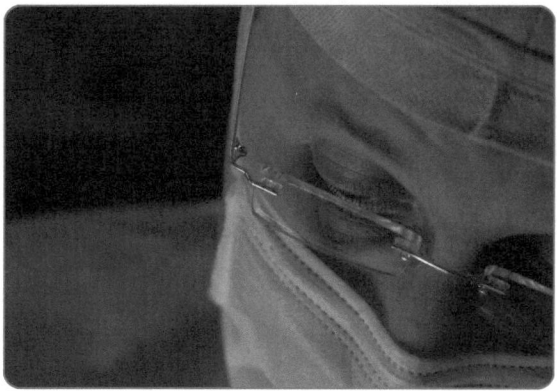

CTR: carpal tunnel release
Her carpal tunnel syndrome will require CTR.

    5. _____ (Abbreviation)

    6. _____

EBL: estimated blood loss
EBL: 200 cc.

    7. _____ (Abbreviation)

    8. _____

EGD: esophagogastroduodenoscopy
EGD revealed no lesions.

    9. _____ (Abbreviation)

   10. _____

II. FILL IN THE BLANK.
Some spaces may require more than one word. Be sure to provide the complete answer. For any question that may have more than one appropriate answer, just choose one.

    1. He had a below-knee _____ performed.

    2. Carpal _____ release was scheduled.

    3. GI performed an _____ .

    4. _____ blood loss was minimal.

    5. An above-_____ amputation was performed at another facility.

III. FILL IN THE BLANK.
Expand the following abbreviations. For any abbreviation that has more than one expansion, just choose one that is appropriate for this lesson.

1. EBL _____   2. AKA _____

3. BKA _____   4. CTR _____

5. EGD _____

I. ENTER ABBREVIATIONS.
Enter the abbreviation and what it stands for.

ET: endotracheal (usually tube)
Anesthesia was general ET tube.

    1. _____ (Abbreviation)

    2. _____

I&D: incision and drainage
He was admitted for I&D of his infected wound.

    3. _____ (Abbreviation)

    4. _____

IJ: internal jugular
The line was placed via a right IJ approach.

    5. _____ (Abbreviation)

    6. _____

IM: intramuscular
IM medicines were administered.

    7. _____ (Abbreviation)

    8. _____

IV: intravenous
He was started on IV antibiotics.

    9. _____ (Abbreviation)

    10. _____

II. FILL IN THE BLANK.
Some spaces may require more than one word. Be sure to provide the complete answer. For any question that may have more than one appropriate answer, just choose one.

    1. For administration of medications, _____ venous line was started.

    2. The administration of intra_____ drugs was ordered.

    3. Anesthesia was per _____ tube.

    4. The catheter was inserted via a left internal _____ approach.

    5. He had an _____ and 6._____ of his infected right knee abscess.

    Expand the following abbreviations. For any abbreviation that has more than one expansion, just choose one that is appropriate for this lesson.

    1. IV_____   2. ET_____

    3. IM_____   4. I&D_____

    5. IJ_____

Surgery – Lesson 3

I. ENTER ABBREVIATIONS.
    Enter the abbreviation and what it stands for.

lap: laparotomy or laparoscopic
Lap cholecystectomy was performed.

    1. _____ (Abbreviation)

    2. _____

LR: lactated Ringer's
1,000 cc LR was administered.

    3. _____ (Abbreviation)

    4. _____

K-wire: Kirschner wire
A K-wire was used for fixation.

    5. _____ (Abbreviation)

    6. _____

NG: nasogastric (usually tube)
An NG tube was inserted.

    7. _____ (Abbreviation)

    8. _____

ORIF: open reduction, internal fixation
He was taken to the OR where ORIF was performed of the ankle fracture.

    9. _____ (Abbreviation)

    10. _____

II. FILL IN THE BLANK.
Some spaces may require more than one word. Be sure to provide the complete answer. For any question that may have more than one appropriate answer, just choose one.

1. Open _____ internal 2._____ of the fracture was performed.

3. A _____ tube was inserted for feedings.

4. _____ wire fixation was utilized.

5. She failed _____ cholecystectomy, and open procedure was undertaken.

6. The patient was administered 1500 cc lactated _____.

III. FILL IN THE BLANK.
Expand the following abbreviations. For any abbreviation that has more than one expansion, just choose one that is appropriate for this lesson.

1. NG_____   2. ORIF _____

3. LR_____   4. K-wire _____

5. lap_____

Surgery – Lesson 4

I. ENTER ABBREVIATIONS.
Enter the abbreviation and what it stands for.

SG: Swan-Ganz (usually catheter)
An SG tube was inserted.

1. _____ (Abbreviation)

2. _____

T&A: tonsillectomy and adenoidectomy
Routine T&A was performed.

3. _____ (Abbreviation)

4. _____

THA: total hip arthroplasty
He was admitted for revision of right THA.

5. _____ (Abbreviation)

6. _____

TKA: total knee arthroplasty
He had a TKA performed on the left five years ago.

    7. _____ (Abbreviation)

    8. _____

TURBT: transurethral resection of the bladder tumor
He had TURBT performed on the second hospital day.

    9. _____ (Abbreviation)

  10. _____

TURP: transurethral resection of the prostate
TURP was performed for BPH.

  11. _____ (Abbreviation)

  12. _____

II. FILL IN THE BLANK.
Some spaces may require more than one word. Be sure to provide the complete answer. For any question that may have more than one appropriate answer, just choose one.

1. A right total knee _____ was performed for degenerative joint disease.

2. _____ resection of the bladder was carried out.

3. A _____ catheter was inserted via the right IJ approach.

4. Transurethral _____ of the prostate was performed by Urology.

5. A revision total _____ arthroplasty was planned.

6. Tonsillectomy and _____ was performed.

III. FILL IN THE BLANK.
Expand the following abbreviations. For any abbreviation that has more than one expansion, just choose one that is appropriate for this lesson.

1. THA_____

2. TURBT_____

3. SG_____

4. TKA_____

5. TURP_____

6. T&A_____

Review: Surgery

I. FILL IN THE BLANK.
Using the word/word parts in the box, enter the appropriate term in the space provided.

1. Incision and _____

2. Swan-_____ catheter

3. Above-knee _____

4. _____-knee amputation

5. Endo_____

6. _____ blood loss

7. Total knee _____

8. _____ wire

9. _____ muscular

10. Intra_____

amputation
arthroplasty
below
drainage
estimated
Ganz
intra
Kirschner
tracheal
venous

II. MATCHING.
Match the word or word part for the appropriate abbreviation expansion. A term may be used more than once.

1. ____ THA – _____ hip arthroplasty

2. ____ TURP – _____ resection of the prostate

3. ____ NG – naso _____ tube

4. ____ T&A – _____ and adenoidectomy

5. ____ ORIF – open _____, internal fixation

6. ____ IM – intra _____

7. ____ I&D – _____ and drainage

8. ____ EGD – esophagogastro _____

9. ____ TURBT – transurethral resection of the bladder _____

10. ____ lap – _____

A. tonsillectomy
B. transurethral
C. duodenoscopy
D. muscular
E. total
F. incision
G. reduction
H. gastric
I. tumor
J. laparotomy

Ancillary Abbreviations – Lesson 1

Following are a number of abbreviations that are not part of any of the previously outlined categories but are important to commit to memory. These are general terms used often in medical reports and you should be able to identify them. Some abbreviations obviously make reference to specific specialties, but they are included here because we have not provided a section for every possible specialty. This is a sort of "catch all" group of abbreviations designed to round out our abbreviations unit.

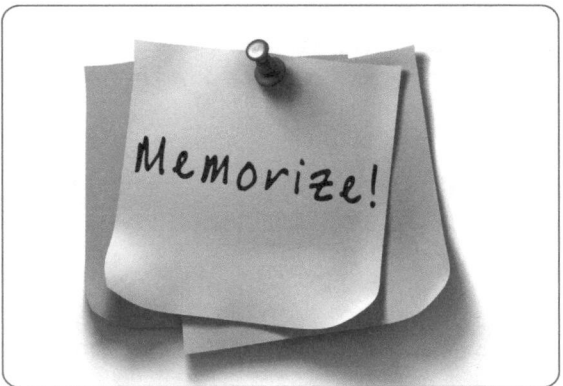

I. **ENTER ABBREVIATIONS.**
    Enter the abbreviation and what it stands for.

ADA: American Dietetic Association
The patient was discharged on ADA diet.

1. _____ (Abbreviation)

2. _____

ADL: activities of daily living
The patient presents to physical therapy having problems with ADLs.

3. _____ (Abbreviation)

4. _____

AMA: against medical advice
The patient signed out AMA.

5. _____ (Abbreviation)

6. _____

Note: AMA also means American Medical Association. The context of the report should make this distinction fairly easy.

ASA: acetylsalicylic acid (aspirin)
He was to take ASA daily for his CAD.

7. _____ (Abbreviation)

8. _____

AVM: arteriovenous malformation
Head CT showed an AVM.

9. _____ (Abbreviation)

10. _____

CLL: chronic lymphocytic leukemia
The primary diagnosis was CLL.

    11. _____ (Abbreviation)

    12. _____

CPAP: continuous positive airway pressure
He was put on CPAP for his sleep apnea.

    13. _____ (Abbreviation)

    14. _____

CPR: cardiopulmonary resuscitation
CPR attempts failed, and the patient was pronounced dead.

    15. _____ (Abbreviation)

    16. _____

II. FILL IN THE BLANK.
Some spaces may require more than one word. Be sure to provide the complete answer. For any question that may have more than one appropriate answer, just choose one.

1. The patient left the hospital _____ medical 2._____ .

3. Diet: low-salt, low-fat American _____ Association diet.

4. He should be able to resume _____ of daily living.

5. _____ malformation was noted.

6. _____ resuscitation attempts failed.

7. The prognosis for his chronic _____ leukemia was poor.

8. The patient could not take _____ acid because of gastrointestinal problems.

9. The continuous _____ pressure helped alleviate his snoring.

III. FILL IN THE BLANK.
Expand the following abbreviations. For any abbreviation that has more than one expansion, just choose one that is appropriate for this lesson.

1. AMA _____   2. CPR _____

3. ADA _____   4. AVM _____

5. ADL _____   6. ASA _____

7. CLL _____

Ancillary Abbreviations – Lesson 2

I. **ENTER ABBREVIATIONS.**
    Enter the abbreviation and what it stands for.

DC: discontinue or discharge
The patient was to DC his medications.
The patient was DC'd after 10 days.

1. _____ (Abbreviation)

2. _____

DNR: DO NOT RESUSCITATE
The patient was counseled and DNR status was confirmed.

3. _____ (Abbreviation)

4. _____

Note that the entire phrase is capitalized. Unless client instructs you otherwise, always type it in caps.

DT: delirium tremens
DTs were noted on presentation at the ER.

5. _____ (Abbreviation)

6. _____

DOB: date of birth
They couldn't find her DOB on her patient chart.

7. _____ (Abbreviation)

8. _____

ESWL: extracorporeal shock-wave lithotripsy
We attempted to destroy the kidney stones with ESWL.

9. _____ (Abbreviation)

10. _____

II. FILL IN THE BLANK.
Some spaces may require more than one word. Be sure to provide the complete answer. For any question that may have more than one appropriate answer, just choose one.

1. With _____ shock-wave 2._____ stones can be removed without surgery.

3. Upon admission her chronic medications were _____.

4. She is a DO NOT _____ status.

5. Her date of _____ is not recorded on the chart.

6. In spite of a long history of alcoholism, he had no record of _____ tremens or blackouts.

III. FILL IN THE BLANK.
Expand the following abbreviations. For any abbreviation that has more than one expansion, just choose one that is appropriate for this lesson.

1. DT _____

2. DNR _____

3. DC _____

4. DOB _____

5. ESWL _____

Ancillary Abbreviations – Lesson 3

I. ENTER ABBREVIATIONS.
Enter the abbreviation and what it stands for.

GE: gastroesophageal
GE reflux is also called heartburn.

1. _____ (Abbreviation)

2. _____

HCTZ: hydrochlorothiazide
HCTZ was part of his high blood pressure control regimen.

3. _____ (Abbreviation)

4. _____

H&P: history and physical
H&P was recorded in the chart.

    5. _____ (Abbreviation)

    6. _____

HPI: history of present illness
For review of systems, see HPI.

    7. _____ (Abbreviation)

    8. _____

II. FILL IN THE BLANK.
Some spaces may require more than one word. Be sure to provide the complete answer. For any question that may have more than one appropriate answer, just choose one.

    1. _____ of present illness as noted above.

    2. There was ulceration at the _____ junction.

    3. _____ has significant side effects in a very few patients.

    4. History and _____ were absent from the chart.

III. FILL IN THE BLANK.
Expand the following abbreviations. For any abbreviation that has more than one expansion, just choose one that is appropriate for this lesson.

    1. HPI _____   2. GE _____

    3. HCTZ _____   4. H&P _____

Ancillary Abbreviations – Lesson 4

I. ENTER ABBREVIATIONS.
Enter the abbreviation and what it stands for.

IOL: intraocular lens
He had an IOL implant O.D. for cataracts.

    1. _____ (Abbreviation)

    2. _____

ITP: idiopathic thrombocytopenic purpura
ITP is characterized by small hemorrhages which may be macular or papular.

3. _____ (Abbreviation)

4. _____

LLL: left lower lobe
The patient has LLL pneumonia.

5. _____ (Abbreviation)

6. _____

LOC: loss of consciousness
Despite head trauma, there was no LOC.

7. _____ (Abbreviation)

8. _____

MDI: metered dose inhaler
The patient was given an Albuterol MDI.

9. _____ (Abbreviation)

10. _____

NKDA: no known drug allergies
Allergies: NKDA.

11. _____ (Abbreviation)

12. _____

II. **FILL IN THE BLANK.**
Some spaces may require more than one word. Be sure to provide the complete answer. For any question that may have more than one appropriate answer, just choose one.

1. She was given an Atrovent metered _____.

2. Idiopathic _____ purpura has such symptoms as easy bruisability.

3. _____ allergies.

4. Loss of _____ was less than one minute.

5. She was admitted for left _____ pneumonia.

6. The _____ lens implant greatly increased her visual acuity in the right eye.

III. **FILL IN THE BLANK.**
Expand the following abbreviations. For any abbreviation that has more than one expansion, just choose one that is appropriate for this lesson.

1. LOC _____   2. IOL _____

3. NKDA _____   4. LLL _____

5. MDI _____   6. ITP _____

Ancillary Abbreviations – Lesson 5

I. **ENTER ABBREVIATIONS.**
Enter the abbreviation and what it stands for.

NPO: nothing by mouth
(NPO is derived from the Latin nil per os.)
She remained NPO on the second postoperative day.

1. _____ (Abbreviation)

2. _____

Can also be written n.p.o. or npo.

Phen-fen: phentermine and fenfluramine
Phen-fen is largely discredited as a weight loss regimen.

3. _____ (Abbreviation)

4. _____

The FDA requested the removal of Phen-fen from the market in 1997. This is also acceptably referred to as fen-phen or Fen-phen. There is acceptable variation to how it is presented.

PND: paroxysmal nocturnal dyspnea
No PND or orthopnea.

5. _____ (Abbreviation)

6. _____

subq: subcutaneous (subcutaneously)
She was injected subq.

7. _____ (Abbreviation)

8. _____

Pronounced sub-Q. Sometimes written subcu.

SOB: shortness of breath
She had severe SOB and was referred to the ER.

   9. _____ (Abbreviation)

   10. _____

TPN: total parenteral nutrition
She was started on TPN while in the hospital.

   11. _____ (Abbreviation)

   12. _____

II. FILL IN THE BLANK.
Some spaces may require more than one word. Be sure to provide the complete answer. For any question that may have more than one appropriate answer, just choose one.

   1. She was injected _____ .

   2. Total _____ nutrition was begun.

   3. She had severe _____ of breath.

   4. _____ by mouth for two days.

   5. No evidence of _____ nocturnal 6._____ .

   7. The patient developed severe heart disease as a result of taking phentermine and

      _____ .

III. FILL IN THE BLANK.
Expand the following abbreviations. For any abbreviation that has more than one expansion, just choose one that is appropriate for this lesson.

   1. NPO _____   2. SOB _____

   3. TPN _____   4. subq _____

   5. PND _____   6. Phen-fen _____

Review: Ancillary Abbreviations

I. FILL IN THE BLANK.
Using the word/word parts in the box, enter the appropriate term in the space provided.

1. against medical _____

2. _____ dose inhaler

3. date of _____

4. total _____

5. _____ of daily living

6. _____ lobe

7. loss of _____

8. _____ of breath

9. cardiopulmonary _____

10. dis_____

activities
advice
birth
consciousness
continue
left lower
metered
parenteral nutrition
resuscitation
shortness

II. MATCHING.
Match the word or word part for the appropriate abbreviation expansion. A term may be used more than once.

1. ____ PND – _____ nocturnal dyspnea

2. ____ NKDA – no known drug _____

3. ____ DT – delirium _____

4. ____ CPAP – continuous positive _____ pressure

5. ____ CLL – chronic _____ leukemia

6. ____ ESWL – _____ shock-wave lithotripsy

7. ____ HCTZ – hydro _____

8. ____ HPI – history of present _____

9. ____ ASA – _____ acid

10. ____ IOL – intra _____ lens

A. lymphocytic
B. tremens
C. airway
D. acetylsalicylic
E. paroxysmal
F. chlorothiazide
G. ocular
H. extracorporeal
I. illness
J. allergies

III. MULTIPLE CHOICE.
Choose the correct word or word part for the abbreviation expansion.

1. ADA – American (◯Diabetic, ◯Dietetic) Association

2. AVM – (◯arteriovenous, ◯arterovenous) malformation

3. ITP – idiopathic thrombocytopenic (◯purpura, ◯purpera)

4. CLL – chronic (◯lymphoma, ◯lymphocytic) leukemia

5. SOB – shortness of (◯breadth, ◯breath)

6. MDI – (◯measured, ◯metered) dose inhaler

7. ADL – activities of daily (◯living, ◯life)

8. DC – (◯discontinue, ◯deliriocremens) .

9. LLL – left lower (◯lobe, ◯lung) .

10. TPN – total (◯parental, ◯parenteral) nutrition

Dangerous Abbreviations

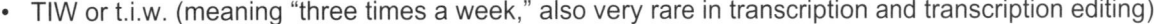

As a word of caution, the use of certain abbreviations is discouraged by hospital accreditation bodies as being "dangerous." So, although they may be listed and used throughout the various components of the course and it is likely you will hear them dictated, your client or employer may instruct you not to use them even when the dictators do. Among these are:

- All the short forms denoting eyes and ears: AS, AD, AU, OS, OD, and OU, with or without periods (spell out the terms, "left ear," "right eye," "both ears," etc.)
- cc (meaning "cubic centimeter." Use mL).
- DC (meaning either discharge or discontinue).
- h.s. (meaning either "at bedtime" or "half-strength," easily confused with each other).
- OD or o.d., or q.o.d. (meaning "once daily," and "every other day," very rare in transcription and transcription editing).
- q.d., q.i.d. (easily confused with one another).
- SC or sub q (for "subcutaneous"; spell out the word).
- TIW or t.i.w. (meaning "three times a week," also very rare in transcription and transcription editing).
- U for "unit" and IU for "international unit."

It is important to be aware of dangerous abbreviations, and we will touch on them again in this training program, especially in the practicum. It is also important to remember that these are not steadfast "rules" of all medical transcription, but health information integrity guidelines put together by accreditation bodies such as

AHDI (Association for Healthcare Documentation Integrity), ISMP (Institute for Safe Medical Practices), and the Joint Commission. This program's practicums contain abbreviations transcribed and dictated in a variety of acceptable ways, ranging from more traditional notations to those correcting for Dangerous Abbreviations.

It is likely that your client or employer will provide instruction on the usage of these and perhaps other abbreviated forms. To learn more about dangerous abbreviations and for a complete list of abbreviations included, perform an online search for "ISMP Dangerous Abbreviations."

Review: Abbreviations

I. **MULTIPLE CHOICE.**
   Mark the following valid or invalid.

1. DBT – deep brachial thrombosis
   - ○ valid
   - ○ invalid

2. SOB – shortness of breath
   - ○ valid
   - ○ invalid

3. SNR – sublingual nitroglycerin relief
   - ○ valid
   - ○ invalid

4. TCL – total cruciate ligament
   - ○ valid
   - ○ invalid

5. LCA – left circumflex artery
   - ○ valid
   - ○ invalid

6. OMB – obtuse marginal branch
   - ○ valid
   - ○ invalid

7. EMA – estimated maternal age
   - ○ valid
   - ○ invalid

8. CMB – complete metabolic blood
   - ○ valid
   - ○ invalid

9. LBC – leftover blood count

○ valid

○ invalid

10. HPI – history of present illness

○ valid

○ invalid

II. MULTIPLE CHOICE.
Choose the appropriate word or word part for the abbreviation expansion.

1. EDC – estimated date of (○confinement, ○conception)

2. TURP – transurethral resection of the (○prostrate, ○prostate)

3. MI – myocardial (○infarction, ○infraction)

4. CVA – costo (○vertebral, ○vertical) angle

5. IVC – (○interior, ○inferior) vena cava

6. COPD – chronic obstructive (○pulmonary, ○pituitary) disease

7. PCL – (○proximal, ○posterior) cruciate ligament

8. TAH-BSO – total abdominal hysterectomy, bilateral (○salpingo-oophorectomy, ○ salpingectomy)

9. ROM – (○rotation, ○rupture) of membranes

10. CHF – (○cardiac, ○congestive) heart failure

11. BPD – biparietal (○diagnosis, ○diameter) test

12. PIP – (○posterior, ○proximal) interphalangeal

13. ORIF – open reduction, (○internal, ○instant) fixation

14. VCUG – voiding (○catheter urogram, ○cystourethrogram)

15. LIMA – (○left, ○lower) internal mammary artery

16. RSV – respiratory (○syndactyly, ○syncytial) virus

17. KUB – kidneys, (○ureters, ○uterus), bladder

18. CVA – cerebrovascular (◯accident, ◯angle)

19. I&D – incision and (◯debridement, ◯drainage)

20. URI – (◯urinary, ◯upper) respiratory infection

III. MATCHING.
Match the word or word part for the appropriate abbreviation expansion. A term may be used more than once.

1. ____ AC – _____ circumference

2. ____ IUGR – _____ growth retardation

3. ____ PTCA – _____ transluminal coronary angioplasty

4. ____ EF – ejection _____

5. ____ AC – acromio _____

6. ____ ADL – activities of daily _____

7. ____ DVT – deep venous _____

8. ____ DJD – degenerative _____ disease

9. ____ TIA – transient ischemic _____

10. ____ TMJ – temporomandibular _____

A. percutaneous
B. thrombosis
C. clavicular
D. joint
E. membrane
F. living
G. abdominal
H. attack
I. fraction
J. intrauterine

IV. MULTIPLE CHOICE.
Choose the best answer.

1. D&C
   ◯ dilatation and curettage
   ◯ dilatation and crushing
   ◯ destruction and curettage
   ◯ destruction and crushing

2. NG
   ◯ nares gastricular
   ◯ nasogenitourinary
   ◯ nasogastrointestine
   ◯ nasogastric

3. TKA

- ○ total knee amputation
- ○ total knee arthroplasty
- ○ top knee amputation
- ○ total knee abscess

4. OR

- ○ outpatient relief
- ○ outpatient room
- ○ operation release
- ○ operating room

5. CPR

- ○ cardiopediatric resuscitation
- ○ cardioproximal resuscitation
- ○ cardiopulmonary resuscitation
- ○ craniopelvic resuscitation

6. PVC

- ○ proximal ventricular contraction
- ○ premature ventricular contraction
- ○ pelvicoventricular contraction
- ○ previous ventricular contraction

7. SLE

- ○ system lupus erythematosus
- ○ systematic lupus erythematosus
- ○ systemic lupus erythematosus
- ○ systematical lupus erythematosus

8. PE

- ○ primary embolism
- ○ pulmonary embolism
- ○ proximal embolism
- ○ percutaneous embolism

9. PDA

○ patent ductus arteriosus
○ patient ductus arteriosus
○ patient ductis arteriosis
○ patented ductus arteriosis

10. MI

○ myocardial infraction
○ miocardial infarction
○ myocardial infarction
○ myocardial infection

Unit 4
Plurals

Plurals – Introduction

There are general as well as specific rules for forming plurals in the English language, and we will cover pluralization of both general words and medical words. Because medical words are, for the most part, of Latin and Greek origins, the rules for pluralization are much more complex. If you are ever in doubt as to how to make a medical word plural, check a medical dictionary or a reputable online medical word resource. If there is no plural form next to the word, then use the basic English language rules.

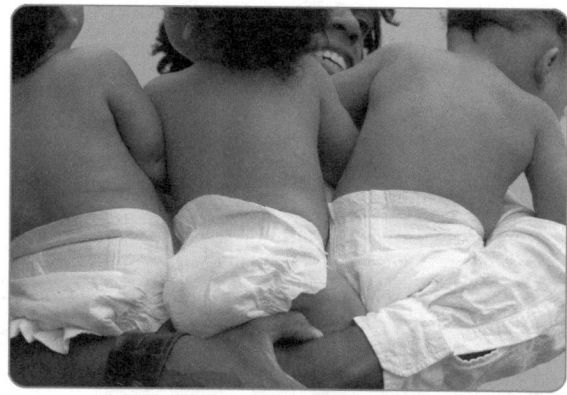

Again, be diligent and verify the accuracy of plural forms. Do not simply trust the way a plural word is dictated as being the correct plural form. A dictator may not know the plural form of a word and may dictate it applying the wrong rules. For example, you learned in the anatomy section that the fingers and toes are called *phalanges*. This is the plural form of the word *phalanx*, which is used when referring to only one finger or toe. However, dictators will often refer to a single finger or toe as a "phalange." You should be aware that this is incorrect, and you need to fix it if your account specifics allow. Your knowledge of the rules governing plurals makes it much easier for you to identify and correct dictator errors.

If you are ever in doubt as to how to make a medical word plural, check a medical dictionary or a reputable online medical word resource.

Plurals – Rules 1—3

There are three basic English rules about forming plurals. You learned these in school and use them in your everyday language. Consequently, they are reviewed here only briefly for your reference.

Plural Rule #1: For most words, simply add an -s to the end of the word.

EXAMPLES: sample = samples, bed = beds, specimen = specimens, pill = pills, doctor = doctors, hospital = hospitals

There is an important exception to Rule #1 that appears often in medical reports. That is for the word *echo*. Although it is a basic word that does not fall into any of the categories shown, it requires an *-es* be added. Thus, the correct plural form of the word *echo* is *echoes*. This can be seen in other English words ending in *o* as well, such as *potato* and *tomato*.

Plural Rule #2: For words ending in -s, -z, -ch, -sh (and nonmedical -x) add an -es to the end of the word.

EXAMPLES: dish = dishes, lunch = lunches, loss = losses, reflex = reflexes

Plural Rule #3: For words ending in -y which are preceded by a consonant, change the -y to an i and add -es. (For words ending in -y preceded by a vowel simply add an -s, i.e., plays, monkeys.)

EXAMPLES: allergy = allergies, anomaly = anomalies, body = bodies, abnormality = abnormalities, party = parties

Enter the correct plural form of the word in the space provided.

1. search _____
2. history _____
3. avulsion _____
4. extremity _____
5. calcification _____
6. church _____
7. cytology _____
8. day _____
9. emergency _____
10. fracture _____
11. duty _____
12. trauma _____
13. boss _____
14. blush _____
15. angiography _____
16. echo _____
17. leukocyte _____
18. stitch _____
19. peduncle _____
20. theology _____

Plurals – Rule 4

Plural Rule #4: *For words ending in -um change the -um to an -a.*

EXAMPLES: antrum = antra, ostium = ostia, velum = vela, ischium = ischia, diverticulum = diverticula.

NOTE: One of life's great certainties is that language constantly changes. Be aware that, although you are learning the standard Latin medical plurals, the fact is that many dictators simply add an *s*. Generally, it is all right to put the word they dictate: *antrums, stromas, ganglions, craniums, leiomyomas*. In addition, as with many grammatical issues, there are exceptions to almost every rule.

I. **FILL IN THE BLANK.**
   Following are words that require use of the above rule for making them plural. In the space provided, enter the plural form of each word.

1. acetabulum _____
2. antrum _____
3. brachium _____
4. capitulum _____
5. cavum _____
6. cilium _____
7. coccidium _____
8. cranium _____
9. diverticulum _____
10. dorsum _____
11. endometrium _____
12. endothelium _____

13. epithelium _____   14. frenulum _____

15. haustrum _____   16. hilum _____

17. infundibulum _____   18. ischium _____

19. labium _____   20. labrum _____

21. mediastinum _____   22. omentum _____

23. ostium _____   24. planum _____

25. pudendum _____   26. retinaculum _____

27. rostrum _____   28. spatium _____

29. spectrum _____   30. speculum _____

31. stratum _____   32. tegmentum _____

33. tentorium _____   34. tuberculum _____

35. reticulum _____

Plurals – Rule 5

Plural Rule #5: For words that end in -a, add an -e.

EXAMPLES: bursa = bursae, lingula = lingulae, uvula = uvulae

There is an important exception to this rule for words ending in -oma or -gma such as stroma. In this instance, add the letters -ta to the end of the word (stromata). Other examples of this are stigma = stigmata, leiomyoma = leiomyomata.

Another exception is in the following two words. These words appear only as plural forms: *adnexa* and *genitalia*. These should be treated as plurals in grammatical usage. "Genitalia are normal." (not "is") There are singular forms, but you will never see or hear them.

I. **FILL IN THE BLANK.**
    Following are words that require use of the above rule for making them plural. In the space provided, enter the plural form of each word.

1. adnexa _____   2. uvula _____

3. fascia _____   4. stoma _____

5. trochlea _____   6. vagina _____

7. medulla _____ 8. vertebra _____

9. condyloma _____ 10. petechia _____

11. vallecula _____ 12. ampulla _____

13. synechia _____ 14. plica _____

15. porta _____ 16. leiomyoma _____

17. stria _____ 18. lingua _____

19. genitalia _____ 20. sequela _____

21. bulla _____ 22. scatoma _____

23. areola _____ 24. conjunctiva _____

25. sella _____ 26. stroma _____

27. vesicula _____ 28. aura _____

29. concha _____ 30. sclera _____

Plurals – Rule 6

Plural Rule #6: For words ending in -us, replace the -us with a single -i.

EXAMPLES: lobus = lobi, tragus = tragi, focus = foci

There are exceptions to this rule as well.

First, there are two words you should memorize, *meatus* and *plexus*. Their plural and singular forms are exactly the same. Grammatically, they are treated as singular forms. "The solar plexus is tender to palpation."

Second, there are three unusual exceptions, all ending in *-us*. These are: *viscus* which becomes *viscera*; *crus* which becomes *crura*; and *corpus* which becomes *corpora*. You should memorize these exceptions.

I. **FILL IN THE BLANK.**
    Following are words that require use of the above rule for making them plural. In the space provided, enter the plural form of each word.

1. stimulus _____ 2. alveolus _____

3. annulus _____ 4. viscus _____

5. malleolus _____ 6. ramus _____

7. meatus _____ 8. truncus _____

9. humerus _____ 10. panniculus _____

11. crus _____ 12. glomerulus _____

13. globus _____ 14. limbus _____

15. vagus _____ 16. uterus _____

17. corpus _____ 18. meniscus _____

19. thrombus _____ 20. fundus _____

21. nevus _____ 22. canaliculus _____

23. plexus _____ 24. bronchus _____

25. calculus _____ 26. sulcus _____

27. bacillus _____ 28. talus _____

29. villus _____ 30. tophus _____

Plurals – Rules 7—8

Plural Rule #7: *For words ending in -en, change the -en to -ina.*

EXAMPLES: foramen = foramina, lumen = lumina

This is an uncommon ending; be sure to note the examples above.

Plural Rule #8: *In words ending in -is, change the -i to an -e.*

EXAMPLES: metastasis = metastases, naris = nares, pelvis = pelves

There are exceptions to this rule as well. These, although uniform, are unusual exceptions and should be memorized individually. They are: *arthritis*, which becomes *arthritides*; *cuspis*, which becomes *cuspides*; and *iris*, which becomes *irides*.

I. **FILL IN THE BLANK.**
    Following are words that require use of the above rules for making them plural. In the space provided, enter the plural form of each word.

1. ankylosis _____ 2. testis _____

3. iris _____ 4. paralysis _____

5. epiphysis _____ 6. diuresis _____

7. arthritis _____ 8. prosthesis _____

9. pubis _____   10. anastomosis _____

11. diaphysis _____   12. metastasis _____

13. cuspis _____   14. synchondrosis _____

15. aponeurosis _____

Plurals – Rule 9

Plural Rule #9: *In words ending in either -ex or -ix, the ending is replaced with -ices.*

*An exception to the rule is the word **reflex**. The only acceptable plural is **reflexes**.*

EXAMPLES: cervix = cervices, apex = apices, vertex = vertices

If any other letter precedes the -x in the word (with the exception of -n), simply replace the -x with -ces.

EXAMPLES: falx = falces, thorax = thoraces

Finally, if the -x is preceded by the letter -n, replace the -x with -ges.

EXAMPLES: pharynx = pharynges, phalanx = phalanges

I. **FILL IN THE BLANK.**
   Following are words that require use of the above rule for making them plural. In the space provided, enter the plural form of each word.

1. appendix _____   2. vortex _____

3. crux _____   4. larynx _____

5. calix _____   6. thorax _____

7. index _____   8. falx _____

9. apex _____   10. matrix _____

11. cicatrix _____   12. phalanx _____

13. varix _____   14. cervix _____

15. vertex _____

Review: Plurals

I. **FILL IN THE BLANK.**
   Enter the correct plural form of the word in the space provided.

1. bronchus _____

2. echo _____

3. labrum _____

4. torus _____

5. adnexa _____

6. lamella _____

7. appendix _____

8. viscus _____

9. branch _____

10. reticulum _____

11. corpus _____

12. tegmentum _____

13. mamma _____

14. condyloma _____

15. chemistry _____

16. fistula _____

17. falx _____

18. arthritis _____

19. panniculus _____

20. cicatrix _____

21. metaphysis _____

22. maxilla _____

23. meatus _____

24. foramen _____

25. speculum _____

26. iris _____

27. humerus _____

28. cervix _____

29. lumen _____

30. spectrum _____

31. apophysis _____

32. sulcus _____

33. phalanx _____

34. malleolus _____

35. pelvis _____

36. ramus _____

37. plexus _____

38. synechia _____

39. prosthesis _____

40. baby _____

Unit 5
Foreign Terms

Foreign Terms – Introduction

As you have already learned, **most medical words come into English from Latin and Greek**. Some of them, like medical plurals, even bring the Latin and/or Greek grammar rules with them. You have been exposed to some of these already:

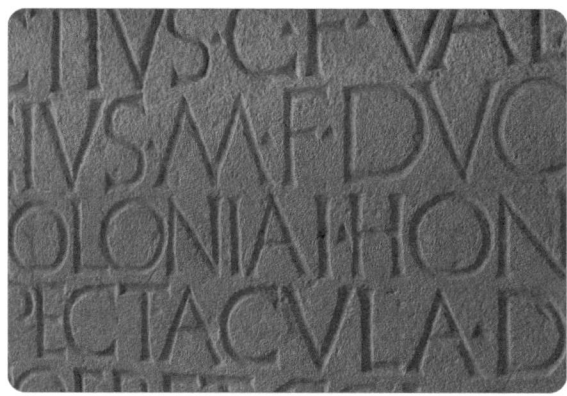

- *condyloma* becomes *condylomata*;
- *adnexus* becomes *adnexa* (in fact, you never see that particular word in the singular);
- *diverticulum* becomes *diverticula*;
- *apex* becomes *apices*;
- *corpus* becomes *corpora*.

Over time, as the words are more widely used, it is likely that the Latin plurals will gradually disappear from common usage: the plural of *ganglion* is equally acceptable as *ganglia* (Latin plural) and *ganglions* (English plural).

For the most part, however, this change has not occurred, so you must learn the rules for plurals, as well as other Latin and Greek forms. Terms like *chondromalacia patellae*, *pruritus vulvae*, and *abruptio placentae* represent the possessive forms of the Latin terms: chondromalacia of the patella, itching of the vulva, and abruption of the placenta.

Fortunately for you, in the workplace where you are using medical terminology, you simply have to be able to identify a term and perhaps make sure it is spelled right, without having to know Latin grammar. (And aren't you glad about that?)

You are exposed to a goodly number of such terms and their definitions in your coursework, and it is important for you to master them. Most of them come, as noted, from the Latin, but some are Greek and others are French.

Some terms are introduced into English usage without undergoing any changes to standardize the term with other medical usage. The medical vocabulary simply includes such terms in their natural non-English form, and they are often pronounced with non-English pronunciations. It is useful for you to learn many of these terms so that you recognize them when you come across them.

One of the tests of a master of medical language is the ability to use words like *en bloc* and *in situ*, knowing what they mean and how to spell them. Not only does the vocabulary of medicine incorporate such terms, but legal vocabulary does as well: *pro bono*, *per annum*, *a priori*, *non sequitur*. These terms, and many others like them, are not at all uncommon in English conversation and writing.

The following lessons introduce you to such terms. These are presented, along with their abbreviations and their definitions, with an occasional instance that demonstrates how they are used. The list is by no means exhaustive, but is intended as a good basic introduction.

Foreign Terms – Lesson 1

Learn these terms, and similar ones should come easy to you when you run across them.

Note: Most of the abbreviated forms of these terms are okay with or without periods: AD or A.D., AS or A.S., OD or O.D., OS or O.S., for example.

I. TERMINOLOGY.

Enter each term in the space provided. Read the definition and description for each term.

1. **addendum** _____

Things to be added. Plural is addenda (or addendums; both are acceptable English usage, but addenda is preferred.).

2. **ad libitum** _____

Shortened to ad lib. According to your pleasure. "The patient is to resume activity ad lib."

3. **auris dextra** _____

A.D., right ear.

4. **auris sinistra** _____

A.S., left ear. Did you know that the word _sinister_ comes from the term that means "left-handed"?

5. **aures utrae** _____

A.U., each ear (often interpreted as "both ears").

6. **bruit(s)** _____

Pronounced broo-ee(s). This is an abnormal vascular sound heard on auscultation during a physical exam. Look it up in your dictionary and you will see that nearly all the different types of bruits are French terms.

7. **cafe au lait spot** _____

This is a skin lesion that is the color of coffee with milk—a distinctive light brown pigment having a macular form. Pronounced "kahFAY o LAY."

8. **coup** _____

A hit or stroke; found in such terms as coup de grace (coo day grawss), coup d'etat (coo day taw), contrecoup (contray-coo—as in a certain kind of brain injury).

9. **cul-de-sac** _____

A blind alley. Usually has reference to the uterine cul-de-sac.

II. FILL IN THE BLANK.

Use terms and not abbreviations in your answers. Some answers may require more than one word to be complete.

1. Coffee-colored. _____

2. Right ear. _____

3. Added thing. _____

4. Blind alley, as the uterus. _____

5. AS or A.S. _____

6. At your pleasure. _____

7. A hit or stroke. _____

8. Both ears or each ear. _____

9. Abnormal sound. _____

Foreign Terms – Lesson 2

I. TERMINOLOGY.
Enter each term in the space provided. Read the definition and description for each term.

1. **en bloc** _____

In one block. Common term in surgery and pathology where a specimen is removed in one piece. It is pronounced "on block." But don't get it wrong by spelling it that way!

2. **en masse** _____

In mass—sometimes refers to one unit, not divided into parts. Pronounced "on mass" or sometimes "on moss."

3. **Gilbert disease** _____

Pronounced zhee-BEAR. An inborn abnormality of liver function.

4. **in ano** _____

About the only place you will ever hear this is in reference to "fistula in ano," which is an abnormal opening near the anus.

5. **in extremis** _____

At the point of death.

6. **in situ** _____

In its original position; in its natural or normal place. "The carcinoma in situ has not spread to surrounding tissues." Very common term in pathology reports.

7. **in toto** _____

As a whole or in the whole, a totality. "The specimen was removed in toto."

II. **FILL IN THE BLANK.**
Use terms and not abbreviations in your answers. Some answers may require more than one word to be complete.

1. Liver function disease. _____

2. Not divided into parts. _____

3. In its original position. _____

4. Totality. _____

5. In a block. _____

6. Near the anus. _____

7. At the point of death. _____

Foreign Terms – Lesson 3

I. **TERMINOLOGY.**
Enter each term in the space provided. Read the definition and description for each term.

1. **oculus dexter** _____

O.D., right eye.

2. **oculus sinister** _____

O.S., left eye.

3. **oculus uterque** _____

O.U., each eye. Again, you will often hear the abbreviations for these terms, but will rarely, if ever, hear the words themselves.

4. **peau d'orange** _____

pronounced "po-dranzh." Literally means "orange peel" and describes the appearance of the skin in certain dermatological conditions.

5. **per** _____

For, through, by. Per diem, by the day. Millimeters per second. Per annum, by the year.

6. **raphe** _____

Pronounced "rah-fay." It is included here because of its unusual pronunciation. Literally the word means "seam" and refers to the line of union between various symmetrical physiologic structures.

7. **Raynaud phenomenon or disease** _____

Pronounced "ray-NO." This is a vascular disorder characterized by intermittent loss of circulation, usually to the extremities.

7. **Raynaud phenomenon or disease** _____

Pronounced "ray-NO." This is a vascular disorder characterized by intermittent loss of circulation, usually to the extremities.

8. **statim** _____

At once, immediately. You will hear this as "stat."

9. **status quo** _____

The existing condition. "There was no change in the patient's status quo."

10. **Virchow-Robin spaces** _____

Pronounced "ver-cow ro-BAN." A perivascular space in the brain in which important immunological functions take place.

II. FILL IN THE BLANK.
Use terms and not abbreviations in your answers. Some answers may require more than one word to be complete.

1. Through or by. _____

2. Immediately. _____

3. Orange peel. _____

4. A seam. _____

5. A space in the brain. _____

6. The existing condition. _____

7. Right eye. _____

8. OS or O.S. _____

9. Vascular phenomenon. _____

10. Each eye or both eyes. _____

Foreign Terms – Lesson 4

The next two lessons introduce you to terms that are used in medication dosage instructions. Of note, much of this information is in the Pharmacology module of this program. These foreign terms are different from most of the ones in this unit because you will rarely, if ever, see them spelled out in context, whatever the context. The abbreviations for them are very commonly used in medical reports, in prescription writing, and in other applications. They are presented here in the classical, formal abbreviation style, such as should be used in legal medical documents (like hospital discharge summaries, consultations, operation reports, etc.). In clinic notes, nurses' notes, other chart notes, prescriptions, and other less formal settings, the periods are often left out of the abbreviated forms: qid, bid, prn, ac, q 4h or q4h, for example. However, in medical transcription they are typically transcribed with the periods.

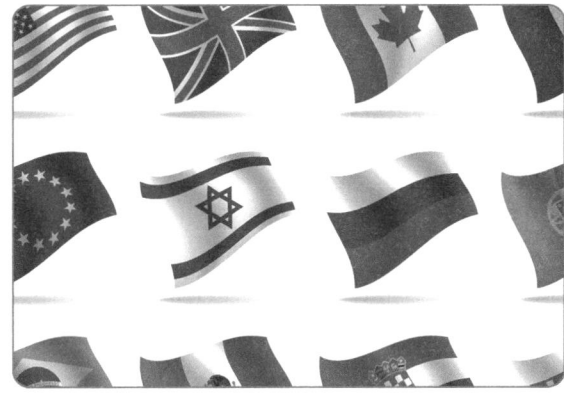

It is important to note that there is considerable variation in the actual dictation of drug dosage instructions and consequently in the transcription of drug dosages as well. Dictators may use the Latin abbreviations, occasional English abbreviations, a mixture of Latin and English abbreviations, or no abbreviations at all (e.g., the dictator may say "q.d," "daily," "q. daily," "once a day," or "every day").

I. TERMINOLOGY.
Enter each term in the space provided. Read the definition and description for each term.

1. **ante cibum** _____

a.c. Before food. "Medication to be taken 40 mg a.c."

2. **ante meridiem** _____

a.m. In the morning. "He will be seen at 10:00 a.m. in the morning"—is totally redundant. Correct it if you see or hear it. The abbreviation a.m. is common in drug dosages. AM is also an acceptable form.

3. **bis in die** _____

b.i.d. Twice a day or twice daily.

4. **die** _____

d. Day. This is the "d" in most abbreviations.

5. **gutta** _____

g.t.t. A drop. Often appears in medication lists in reference to eardrops or eyedrops.

6. **hora** _____

h. Hour. "Amoxicillin 500 mg q.4h. or q. 4 h."

7. **hora somni** _____

h.s. At bedtime (literally the hour of sleep). "She was to take her Elavil q.h.s."

8. **per os** _____

By mouth. "Lasix 40 p.o. q.d."

II. FILL IN THE BLANK.
Enter the English translation of the following terms. Some answers may require more than one word to be complete.

1. hora _____   2. b.i.d. _____

3. p.o. _____   4. h.s. _____

5. a.c. _____   6. die _____

7. gutta _____   8. a.m. _____

Foreign Terms – Lesson 5

I. TERMINOLOGY.
Enter each term in the space provided. Read the definition and description for each term.

1. **post meridiem** _____

p.m. Afternoon, or between noon and midnight.

2. **pro re nata** _____

p.r.n. As needed. "Tylenol 325 mg q.4 h. p.r.n. pain."

3. **quaque die** _____

q.d. Every day.

4. **quaque hora** _____

q.h. Every hour.

5. **quaque secunda hora** _____

Abbreviated q.2 h. This means every 2 hours.

6. **quaque tertia hora** _____

q.3 h. Every 3 hours.

7. **quaque quarta hora** _____

q.4 h. Every 4 hours.

8. **quaque sex hora** _____

q.6 h. Every 6 hours.

9. **quaque octa hora** _____

q.8 h. Every 8 hours.

10. **quater in die** _____

q.i.d. Four times a day.

11. **ter in die** _____

t.i.d. Three times a day.

II. **FILL IN THE BLANK.**
   Expand the following abbreviations. Expand the abbreviated forms to their English equivalent or use the English term for the Latin word.

1. p.m. _____   2. t.i.d. _____

3. pro re nata _____   4. q.i.d. _____

5. q.2h. _____   6. q.d. _____

7. quaque hora _____   8. quaque _____

Review: Foreign Terms

I. **MATCHING.**
   Match the correct term to the definition.

1. ____ in its original position
2. ____ at once
3. ____ abnormal vascular heart sounds
4. ____ by mouth
5. ____ according to your pleasure
6. ____ before food
7. ____ for, through, by
8. ____ every day
9. ____ at bedtime
10. ____ both eyes
11. ____ in one block
12. ____ things to be added
13. ____ three times a day
14. ____ left ear
15. ____ twice a day
16. ____ existing condition
17. ____ at the point of death
18. ____ every 6 hours
19. ____ blind alley
20. ____ referring to one unit

A. p.o. (per os)
B. in extremis
C. t.i.d.
D. in situ
E. per
F. stat
G. a.c.
H. b.i.d.
I. OU
J. bruit
K. h.s.
L. AS
M. q.d.
N. cul-de-sac
O. status quo
P. addendum
Q. en bloc
R. en masse
S. ad lib
T. q.6 h.

Unit 6
Slang and Jargon

Slang and Jargon – Introduction

Slang is the use of informal words and expressions that are not considered standard language, and **jargon** includes special words and expressions typically used by a particular profession. Both slang and jargon are frequently seen in medical transcription, and we hardly even recognize them as such because they have become so commonplace. While abbreviated or shortened forms of terms are often acceptable, the same thing is not necessarily true of slang. In formal medical documents it is typically best to avoid slang terms and phrases unless the meaning cannot be determined otherwise (which is a very rare occurrence) or when they more accurately communicate the meaning (also a rare occurrence).

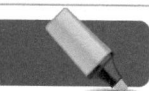
Notwithstanding the above, in some types of medical reports, such as clinic notes and nurses' notes, many slang and jargon terms are acceptable. Simple shortened forms are even more widely acceptable.

Reasons for avoiding the use of slang and jargon are as follows:

1. Expanding the terms allows for more accurate documentation and greater ease of both spoken and written comprehension.
2. Many medical reports are legal documents, and they should be comprehensible to judges and juries.
3. Since patients have the right to review their medical charts, their reports should be written in a language they can understand rather than in medical code.
4. The parents of children under medical care must be able to understand the language in the reports concerning their children.

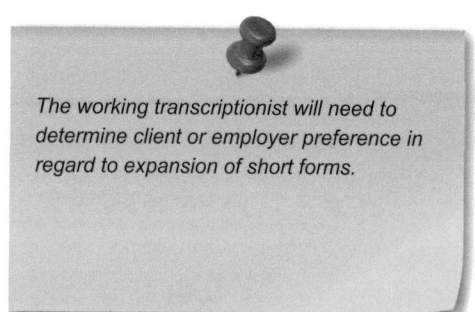

The working transcriptionist will need to determine client or employer preference in regard to expansion of short forms.

The footnotes in the practicums will provide a good deal of information on when and where it is acceptable to use the short forms that are dictated.

Slang and Jargon – Lesson 1

I. **TERMINOLOGY.**
   Enter the formal term in the space provided. Read the definition and description for each term.

   1. **a-fib, A-fib, or AFib** _____
   Atrial fibrillation (a severe cardiac arrhythmia).

   2. **alk phos** _____
   Alkaline phosphatase (a lab value for a chemical in the blood).

   3. **appy** _____
   Appendectomy or appendicitis (excision of the appendix or infection/inflammation of the appendix).

   4. **bicarb** _____
   Bicarbonate (one of the electrolytes, with sodium, potassium, and chloride).

5. **bili** _____

Bilirubin (a lab value for liver function testing).

6. **CBC with diff** _____

CBC (complete blood count) with differential (the percentages of different types of white cells in the blood).

7. **caps** _____

Capsules (a form of medications).

8. **cath** _____

Catheter or catheterization (a tube or the placement of tubes in the body).

9. **chemo** _____

Chemotherapy (treatment with chemical compounds, usually referring to cancer regimens).

10. **chole** _____

Cholecystectomy (excision of the gallbladder).

II. **MATCHING.**
   Match the correct term to the definition.

1. ____ A tube or the placement of tubes in the body.

2. ____ A severe cardiac arrhythmia.

3. ____ Excision of the appendix or inflammation of the appendix.

4. ____ Treatment with chemical compounds.

5. ____ A chemical in the blood.

6. ____ Excision of the gallbladder.

7. ____ A lab value for liver function.

8. ____ A form of medication.

9. ____ Percentages of different types of white blood cells.

10. ____ One of the electrolytes.

A. cholecystectomy
B. chemotherapy
C. complete blood count with differential
D. atrial fibrillation
E. bicarbonate
F. catheter or catheterization
G. appendectomy or appendicitis
H. bilirubin
I. alkaline phosphatase
J. capsules

Slang and Jargon – Lesson 2

I. TERMINOLOGY.
Enter the formal term in the space provided. Read the definition and description for each term.

1. **crit** _____

Hematocrit (test for packed red cells in the blood).

2. **DC** _____

Discontinue or discharge, past tense DC'd, sometimes dc/dc'd (acceptable in a clinic or nurse's note but not in a formal document).

3. **detox** _____

Detoxification (treatment for acute alcohol abuse or other drug overuse).

4. **dig** _____

Digoxin or digitalis; pronounced with a short i and g sounding like j (medication for cardiac problems).

5. **dip sesta** _____

Dipyridamole sestamibi (a nuclear x-ray exam).

6. **double J stent** _____

JJ stent (a surgical device for keeping tubes in place).

7. **echo** _____

Echocardiogram (recording of heart function by analyzing sound waves).

8. **eos** _____

Eosinophils (white blood cells that are part of the CBC with differential).

9. **exam** _____

Examination (evaluation, as in physical examination or Mental Status Examination).

10. **flex sig** _____

Flexible sigmoidoscopy (inspection of the sigmoid, the S-shaped lower portion of the colon, with a flexible endoscopic instrument).

II. MATCHING.
Match the correct term to the definition.

1. ___ Treatment for acute alcohol abuse or other drug overuse

2. ___ White blood cells

3. ___ Evaluation

4. ___ Inspection of the sigmoid with a flexible endoscopic instrument

5. ___ Recording of heart function by analyzing sound waves

6. ___ DC—acceptable in a nurse's note

7. ___ Medication for cardiac problems

8. ___ Surgical device for keeping tubes in place

9. ___ A nuclear x-ray exam

10. ___ A test for packed red blood cells

A. flexible sigmoidoscopy
B. dipyridamole sestamibi
C. digoxin or digitalis
D. eosinophils
E. detoxification
F. JJ stent
G. hematocrit
H. examination
I. discontinue or discharge
J. echocardiogram

Slang and Jargon – Lesson 3

I. TERMINOLOGY.
Enter the formal term in the space provided. Read the definition and description for each term.

1. **Foley** _____

Foley catheter (a catheter commonly used during surgical procedures for draining urine from the bladder).

2. **HCTZ** _____

Hydrochlorothiazide (a medication for the control of hypertension and edema).

3. **hem/onc** _____

Hematology/oncology (the medical specialty that deals with cancer and blood problems).

4. **hep C (A, B)** _____

Hepatitis C (A, B) (liver disease characterized by infection and inflammation).

5. **K** _____

Potassium (the chemical symbol for the element potassium. This is an acceptable usage.)

6. **KCl** _____

Potassium chloride (the chemical formula for potassium chloride; it is often given to cardiac patients whose potassium is depleted by diuretic medications, such as Lasix. This is an acceptable usage.)

7. **lac** _____

Laceration (a cut produced by trauma).

8. **lymphs** _____

Lymphocytes (another type of white blood cell included in the CBC with differential).

9. **lytes** _____

Electrolytes (usually sodium, potassium, chloride, and bicarbonate; they are blood chemistries evaluated in laboratory studies).

10. **mag** _____

Magnesium (a chemical in the blood, also a medication given for some medical conditions, such as alcohol overdose).

II. **MATCHING.**
   Match the correct term to the definition.

1. ____ Liver disease characterized by infection and inflammation.

2. ____ A catheter commonly used during surgical procedures for draining urine from the bladder.

3. ____ Sodium, potassium, chloride, and bicarbonate, blood chemistries evaluated in laboratory studies.

4. ____ A cut produced by trauma.

5. ____ A chemical in the blood, also a medication given for some medical conditions, such as alcohol overdose.

6. ____ The expanded name for the chemical KCl.

7. ____ The medical specialty that deals with cancer and blood problems.

8. ____ Another type of white blood cell included in the CBC with differential.

9. ____ K is the chemical symbol for this element.

10. ____ A medication for the control of hypertension and edema.

A. laceration
B. potassium
C. hepatitis
D. hematology and oncology
E. Foley catheter
F. hydrochlorothiazide
G. potassium chloride
H. electrolytes
I. lymphocytes
J. magnesium

Slang and Jargon – Lesson 4

I. TERMINOLOGY.
   Enter the formal term in the space provided. Read the definition and description for each term.

1. **meds** _____

Medications (drugs given to patients; pharmacopeia).

2. **mets** _____

Metastases, singular met/metastasis (the spread of malignant neoplasm—cancer—from the primary site to one or more secondary sites).

3. **migs** _____

Milligrams, written as mg (metric unit of measurement, the most common form of drug dosage).

4. **mikes** _____

Micrograms, written as mcg (metric unit of measurement smaller than the milligram, also used in some drug dosages).

5. **monos** _____

Monocytes (white blood cells that are a part of the CBC with differential).

6. **nebs** _____

Nebulizers (an aerated form of medications given for pulmonary problems such as asthma).

7. **neuro** _____

Neurological or neurology (referring to the medical specialty or to the part of the physical exam that evaluates neurologic or central nervous system function).

8. **neuropsych** _____

Neuropsychiatric or neuropsychiatry (pertaining to the study of the combination of neurology and psychiatry—often related, since both study brain function).

9. **O2 sat** _____

Oxygen saturation (the amount of oxygen present in the blood; measured by pulse oximetry).

10. **path** _____

Pathology (the study of the essential nature of disease, particularly as it relates to changes in tissues, organs, etc. Also the cause of disease).

Match the definition to the appropriate term.

1. ____ The amount of oxygen present in the blood.

2. ____ Metric units of measurement, the most common form of drug dosage.

3. ____ The study of the essential nature of disease.

4. ____ An aerated form of medications given for pulmonary problems such as asthma.

5. ____ Pertaining to the study of two related medical specialties.

6. ____ Drugs.

7. ____ Metric unit of measurement smaller than the milligram.

8. ____ The spread of cancer from a primary to a secondary site.

9. ____ A part of the physical examination or the study of nerve function.

10. ____ A type of white blood cell.

A. pathology
B. nebulizers
C. medications
D. micrograms
E. metastases
F. monocytes
G. oxygen saturation
H. milligrams
I. neuropsychiatric
J. neurology or neurological

Slang and Jargon – Lesson 5

I. TERMINOLOGY.

Enter the formal term in the space provided. Read the definition and description for each term.

1. **perf** _____

Perforation (a hole, as in a perforated eardrum or perforated bowel).

2. **preop** _____

Preoperative (before an operation). Occasionally, but rarely, a dictator will use the term "preopped" (alternative spelling "preopp'd"). This is not really a short form for anything that can reasonably be expanded without rewriting the sentence. It is an example of a slang/jargon term that "more accurately communicates meaning" than any possible expansion of it would.

3. **postop** _____

Postoperative (after an operation).

4. **prepped** _____

Prepared (a short form commonly used in surgical reports; e.g., "The patient was prepped and draped").

5. **psych** _____

Psychiatry, psychology (the specialties that address the mind and mental processes).

6. **pulse ox** _____

Pulse oximetry (the process of determining oxygen saturation by use of machine measurements).

7. **regurg** _____

Regurgitation (flow in the opposite direction from normal, as in vomiting stomach contents or backward flow of the blood through vascular structures).

8. **rehab** _____

Rehabilitation (the process of restoring normal form and function after injury or illness by means of physical, psychosocial, vocational, or recreational activities).

9. **sat** _____

Saturation (a measure of the degree to which oxygen is bound to the hemoglobin in the blood; it is given as a percentage, and reflects pulmonary function).

II. **MATCHING.**
   Match the correct term to the definition.

1. ____ The process of restoring normal form and function.

2. ____ The means of measuring oxygen saturation.

3. ____ The specialties that address the mind and mental processes.

4. ____ Before an operation.

5. ____ The degree to which oxygen in the blood is bound to hemoglobin.

6. ____ Short form commonly used in surgical reports with "draped."

7. ____ Following surgery.

8. ____ Flow in the opposite direction from normal.

9. ____ A hole.

A. preoperative
B. psychology/psychiatry
C. postoperative
D. regurgitation
E. saturation
F. pulse oximetry
G. prepared
H. rehabilitation
I. perforation

Slang and Jargon – Lesson 6

I. **TERMINOLOGY.**
Enter the formal term in the space provided. Read the definition and description for each term.

1. **sed rate** _____

Sedimentation rate (a laboratory value related to the action of red blood cells).

2. **segs** _____

Segmented neutrophils (white blood cells that are part of the CBC differential).

3. **t. bili** _____

Total bilirubin (a bile pigment that is measured in liver function studies).

4. **tabs** _____

Tablets (a form of medication, pills).

5. **triple A** _____

Abdominal aortic aneurysm (AAA, a cardiovascular anomaly).

6. **V-tach** _____

Ventricular tachycardia (an increased ventricular heart rate).

7. **voc rehab** _____

Vocational rehabilitation (rehabilitation for those who need to retrain in a former or new vocation due to illness or injury).

II. MATCHING.
Match the correct term to the definition.

1. ____ An increased ventricular heart rate.

2. ____ Retraining for a new or former vocation.

3. ____ A laboratory value related to the action of red blood cells.

4. ____ White blood cells that are part of the CBC differential.

5. ____ A form of medication.

6. ____ A cardiovascular anomaly of the aorta.

7. ____ A bile pigment measured in liver function studies.

A. sedimentation rate
B. total bilirubin
C. abdominal aortic aneurysm
D. ventricular tachycardia
E. segmented neutrophils
F. vocational rehabilitation
G. tablets

Review: Slang and Jargon

I. FILL IN THE BLANK.
For each bold slang term, enter the formal term in the space provided.

1. The patient was told to take 4 **caps** _____ a day.

2. A followup **flex sig** _____ will be scheduled.

3. The patient was started on **nebs** _____ .

4. His **O2 sat** _____ was 98% on room air.

5. The wound was **prepped** _____ and draped in sterile fashion.

6. Her **dig** _____ level was checked and was found to be normal.

7. Past surgical history is positive for **appy** _____ in 2001.

8. Patient was found to be in **AFib** _____ and was subsequently cardioverted.

9. The radiograph showed **mets** _____ to the liver.

10. She was taken to the **cath** _____ lab.

II. FILL IN THE BLANK.
Enter the complete formal word in the blank provided.

1. crit _____

2. bicarb _____

3. exam _____

4. migs _____

5. lac _____

6. mag _____

7. perf _____

8. mikes _____

9. regurg _____

10. voc rehab _____

Answer Key

Word Differentiation

Word Differentiation – Lesson 1

I. MATCHING.
1. K. toward the center
3. F. expression of emotion
5. L. an adenoma
7. B. to agree to
9. I. away from the center
11. D. productive of results

2. A. a misleading image
4. G. to leave out
6. J. the result or outcome
8. E. the avoidance of
10. C. disease of the glands
12. H. arising from emotions

II. MULTIPLE CHOICE.
1. accept
3. delusions
5. Effective
7. afferent
9. adenocyst
11. affective
13. alluding

2. affected
4. except
6. effects
8. allusions
10. elusion
12. adenosis
14. eluting

Word Differentiation – Lesson 2

I. MATCHING.
1. H. serous fluid in the abdomen
3. A. line revolved about
5. D. wasting away
7. B. acid-forming
9. M. assisting device
11. L. pertaining to allergies
13. N. person who assists

2. I. involuntary discharge of urine
4. F. excision of arterial plaque
6. J. not poisonous
8. C. displaced
10. E. retention of urine
12. K. lacking strength
14. G. to get at

II. MULTIPLE CHOICE.
1. ascitic
3. enuresis
5. acidic
7. atherectomy
9. access
11. aid
13. attain

2. arthrectomy
4. ectopic
6. anuresis
8. atony
10. atoxic
12. aide
14. obtained

Word Differentiation – Lesson 3

I. MATCHING.
1. B. pertaining to the arm
3. A. pertaining to the ear
5. C. medicinal mass
7. I. pertaining to the mouth
9. G. resembling fish gills
11. D. hard

2. K. bulb-like
4. H. air passage in the lungs
6. J. localized hyperplasia of the epidermis
8. F. characterized by large vesicle
10. E. enlargement

II. MULTIPLE CHOICE.

1. bolus
2. branchial
3. oral
4. bulbous
5. brachial
6. aural
7. callus
8. bullous
9. bulbus
10. bronchial
11. avulsion
12. evulsions

Word Differentiation – Lesson 4

I. MATCHING.

1. J. canal formation
2. I. layer of grey matter
3. H. direction of progress
4. G. contraction
5. C. milky fluid
6. D. rough/harsh
7. F. cannula insertion
8. E. near the ear
9. B. approximation
10. A. neck artery

II. MULTIPLE CHOICE.

1. coarse
2. cannulization
3. parotid
4. claustrum
5. Carotid
6. canalization
7. course
8. coaptation
9. colostrum
10. coarctation

Word Differentiation – Lesson 5

I. MATCHING.

1. B. beak-shaped
2. I. the heart
3. K. study of cells
4. A. flattering remark
5. H. center
6. J. moral indicator
7. D. coating of the eye
8. F. accessory
9. E. awake and alert
10. C. military division
11. G. knowledge of nutrition

II. MULTIPLE CHOICE.

1. Corps
2. complementary
3. coracoid
4. conscious
5. Cytology
6. compliments
7. core
8. choroid
9. Cor
10. conscience

Word Differentiation – Lesson 6

I. MATCHING.

1. I. material for coloring
2. F. to draw out
3. H. abnormal development
4. G. illegal
5. J. repetition of sound
6. B. to stop living
7. E. impairment of speech
8. K. showing good judgment
9. A. difficulty swallowing
10. C. plural echocardiogram
11. D. individually distinct

II. MULTIPLE CHOICE.

1. discrete
2. elicit
3. dye
4. dysphagia
5. echos
6. illicit
7. die
8. dysphasia
9. echoes
10. discreet
11. dysplasia

Word Differentiation – Lesson 7

I. MATCHING.

1. H. increase of symptoms
2. D. closure of wound
3. C. removal of a nerve
4. J. nerve distribution
5. F. excrement
6. B. being irritated
7. G. fibrous tissue
8. E. barium injection
9. I. expression of face
10. A. pertaining to the face

II. MULTIPLE CHOICE.

1. feces
2. enervation
3. fascial
4. exacerbation
5. enterocleisis
6. Innervation
7. facies
8. enteroclysis
9. exasperation
10. facial

Review: Lessons 1—7

I. MATCHING.

1. M. exacerbation
2. C. feces
3. I. compliment
4. K. conscience
5. J. callus
6. H. enterocleisis
7. F. dysphasia
8. Y. enuresis
9. Q. innervation
10. D. dysphagia
11. L. coarse
12. G. efferent
13. O. parotid
14. R. enervation
15. S. atonic
16. A. discreet
17. X. allusion
18. V. cannulization
19. N. accept
20. Z. afferent

II. MULTIPLE CHOICE.

1. exacerbated
2. facial
3. echoes
4. cor
5. affect
6. allusion
7. adenosis
8. ascitic
9. bronchial
10. coaptation

Word Differentiation – Lesson 8

I. MATCHING.

1. F. pertaining to excrement
2. D. at the bottom
3. H. albuminoid substance
4. I. sac in the spine
5. K. uniform quality
6. J. a bending
7. B. sharing a common ancestor
8. E. a muscle flexing a joint
9. C. pertaining to the cecum
10. A. glassy or transparent
11. G. caused by a fungus

1. fundal
2. homogeneous
3. flexure
4. fecal
5. hyaline
6. thecal
7. flexor
8. homogeneous
9. cecal
10. fungal

Word Differentiation – Lesson 9

I. MATCHING.

1. I. enter drop by drop
2. J. leading or bringing in
3. E. rounded process
4. G. to establish in place
5. H. within a cavity
6. B. hip bone
7. A. auditory ossicle
8. F. inducing anesthesia
9. D. portion of small intestine
10. C. within the eye

II. MULTIPLE CHOICE.

1. instillation
2. malleolus
3. ilium
4. induction
5. malleus
6. ileo-
7. installed
8. intralocular
9. introduction
10. intraocular

Word Differentiation – Lesson 10

I. MATCHING.

1. J. pertaining to a door
2. I. free slime
3. F. spread of disease
4. H. bony, osseous
5. G. resembling mucus
6. A. mediastinal operation
7. D. part of the long bone
8. E. cutting through the sternum
9. B. pertaining to the mind
10. C. a fold of peritoneum (adj.)

II. MULTIPLE CHOICE.

1. metaphysis
2. mucus
3. ostial
4. median sternotomy
5. mucous
6. mental
7. metastasis
8. osteal
9. mediastinotomy
10. omentum

Word Differentiation – Lesson 11

I. MATCHING.

1. D. simple
2. G. continue
3. I. serous membrane/abdomen
4. H. fibular
5. C. to go in front of
6. A. area between the thighs
7. J. a straight surface
8. E. injection by alternate route
9. F. pertaining to the perineum
10. B. pertaining to parents

II. MULTIPLE CHOICE.

1. peritoneum
2. proceed
3. peroneal
4. plane
5. parenteral
6. plain
7. preceded
8. parental
9. perineum

Word Differentiation – Lesson 12

I. MATCHING.

1. B. male gland
2. E. abundance
3. M. vocal sound
4. I. pouring over or through
5. K. strictly regulated activity
6. C. involuntary action
7. H. where one lives
8. J. backward flow
9. D. lying horizontal
10. F. military unit
11. L. being thrust forward
12. G. artificial part
13. A. relating to a male gland

II. MULTIPLE CHOICE.

1. perfusion
2. regimen
3. prostate
4. reflexes
5. protrusion
6. prostrate
7. residents
8. prostatic
9. resonance
10. regiment
11. prosthetic
12. reflux

Word Differentiation – Lesson 13

I. MATCHING.

1. F. organic compound
2. G. seeing
3. J. not a real word
4. C. a location
5. D. path
6. I. deep membranous layer
7. H. a region
8. A. the lowermost portion
9. B. nonmetallic element
10. E. channel

II. MULTIPLE CHOICE.

1. route
2. site
3. Scarpa's
4. silicone
5. sight
6. root
7. tract
8. silicon
9. tracked

Word Differentiation – Lesson 14

I. MATCHING.

1. G. towards the tongue
2. D. summit or top
3. C. hook-shaped (adj.)
4. E. used for ulcers
5. K. thick and slow-flowing
6. I. pertaining to the nails
7. A. between the chest and hips
8. B. used for anxiety
9. F. gradual loss or decay
10. H. a whorled design
11. J. large organ

II. MULTIPLE CHOICE.

1. vortex
2. Zantac
3. sublingually
4. vertex
5. wasting
6. Xanax
7. subungual
8. waist
9. uncal
10. viscus
11. viscous

Review: Lessons 8—14

I. MATCHING.

1. G. intraocular
2. R. hyaline
3. H. residents
4. E. site
5. P. ungual
6. Y. peroneal
7. J. prostrate
8. B. flexor
9. O. profusion
10. K. plain
11. U. prostate
12. Z. sight
13. Q. residence
14. S. uncal
15. F. proceed
16. M. osteal
17. T. track
18. D. perfusion
19. L. perineal
20. N. reflux

II. MULTIPLE CHOICE.

1. site
2. tracked
3. viscous
4. protrusion
5. regimen
6. preceded
7. plain
8. mucus
9. fungal
10. ostial

Abbreviations

Diseases and Syndromes – Lesson 1

II. FILL IN THE BLANK.

1. respiratory
2. syndrome
3. acquired
4. deficiency
5. hypertrophy
6. lymphocytic OR lymphoblastic
7. aneurysm

III. FILL IN THE BLANK.

1. benign prostatic hypertrophy OR benign prostatic hyperplasia
2. acquired immune deficiency syndrome OR acquired immunodeficiency syndrome
3. abdominal aortic aneurysm
4. acute lymphocytic leukemia OR acute lymphoblastic leukemia
5. adult respiratory distress syndrome

Diseases and Syndromes – Lesson 2

II. FILL IN THE BLANK.

1. carcinoma
2. chronic obstructive
3. congestive
4. cystic
5. cerebrovascular
6. megalovirus

III. FILL IN THE BLANK.

1. cytomegalovirus
2. chronic obstructive pulmonary disease
3. congestive heart failure
4. carcinoma (cancer) OR cancer (carcinoma)
5. cerebrovascular accident
6. cystic fibrosis

Diseases and Syndromes – Lesson 3

II. FILL IN THE BLANK.
1. idiopathic
2. hyperostosis
3. thrombosis
4. Fibrocystic
5. mellitus
6. degenerative

III. FILL IN THE BLANK.
1. deep venous thrombosis OR deep vein thrombosis
2. diabetes mellitus
3. degenerative joint disease
4. diffuse idiopathic skeletal hyperostosis
5. fibrocystic disease

Diseases and Syndromes – Lesson 4

II. FILL IN THE BLANK.
1. reflux
2. herniated
3. pulposus
4. interstitial
5. insulin-dependent
6. hyaline

III. FILL IN THE BLANK.
1. hyaline membrane disease
2. gastroesophageal reflux disease
3. insulin-dependent diabetes mellitus
4. herniated nucleus pulposus
5. interstitial lung disease

Diseases and Syndromes – Lesson 5

II. FILL IN THE BLANK.
1. sclerosis
2. rheumatoid
3. dystrophy
4. syncytial
5. post-traumatic

III. FILL IN THE BLANK.
1. multiple sclerosis
2. post-traumatic stress disorder
3. respiratory syncytial virus
4. rheumatoid arthritis
5. reflex sympathetic dystrophy

Diseases and Syndromes – Lesson 6

II. FILL IN THE BLANK.
1. respiratory
2. systemic
3. erythematosus
4. ischemic attack
5. urinary
6. infection
7. sudden
8. syndrome

III. FILL IN THE BLANK.
1. transient ischemic attack
2. urinary tract infection
3. systemic lupus erythematosus
4. upper respiratory infection
5. sudden infant death syndrome

Review: Diseases and Syndromes

I. FILL IN THE BLANK.

1. joint
2. cerebro
3. obstructive pulmonary
4. death syndrome
5. transient
6. failure
7. respiratory
8. venous thrombosis
9. urinary
10. idiopathic skeletal

II. MATCHING.

1. G. infection
2. H. arthritis
3. A. cytomegalo
4. F. mellitus
5. J. membrane
6. B. syncytial
7. I. stress
8. C. thrombosis
9. D. carcinoma
10. E. transient

III. MULTIPLE CHOICE.

1. erythematosus
2. cystic
3. sympathetic
4. pulposus
5. reflux
6. interstitial
7. congestive
8. disease
9. multiple
10. cystic

Rooms – Lesson 1

II. FILL IN THE BLANK.

1. intensive care unit
2. emergency room
3. operating room
4. pediatric intensive care unit
5. neonatal intensive care unit
6. coronary care unit
7. surgical intensive care unit

Departments – Lesson 2

II. FILL IN THE BLANK.

1. gynecology
2. obstetrics
3. ears, nose, and throat
4. gastroenterology
5. physical therapy
6. occupational therapy

Weights and Measurements – Lesson 1

II. FILL IN THE BLANK.

1. decibel OR dB
2. centimeter
3. centigray
4. deciliter OR dL
5. centimeter OR cm

III. FILL IN THE BLANK.

1. decibel
2. cubic centimeter
3. centigray
4. deciliter
5. centimeter

Weights and Measurements – Lesson 2

II. FILL IN THE BLANK.
1. g OR gram
2. Hz OR hertz
3. L OR liter
4. mCi OR millicurie
5. mEq OR milliequivalent

III. FILL IN THE BLANK.
1. liter
2. milliequivalent
3. hertz
4. gram
5. millicurie

Weights and Measurements – Lesson 3

II. FILL IN THE BLANK.
1. mg OR milligram
2. mGy OR milligray
3. mHz OR megahertz
4. mL OR milliliter
5. mm OR millimeter

III. FILL IN THE BLANK.
1. milliliter
2. millimeter
3. milligray
4. milligram
5. megahertz

Weights and Measurements – Lesson 4

II. FILL IN THE BLANK.
1. mercury
2. mmol OR millimole
3. msec OR ms
4. meters
5. second
6. meters
7. squared
8. nanometer
9. oz OR ounce

III. FILL IN THE BLANK.
1. nanometer
2. meters per second
3. ounce
4. millimole
5. millimeters of mercury
6. mL OR millisecond
7. mm OR meters per second squared

Review: Weights and Measurements

I. MATCHING.
1. D. Hz
2. I. cGy
3. B. mEq
4. A. ml
5. J. nm
6. G. oz
7. H. L
8. F. mg
9. E. g
10. C. mCi

II. FILL IN THE BLANK.
1. deciliter
2. megahertz
3. cubic centimeter
4. millisecond
5. millimeter
6. meters per second
7. milligray
8. centimeter

9. millimole
11. decibel
13. meters per second squared

10. hertz
12. millimeters of mercury

Cardiology – Lesson 1

II. FILL IN THE BLANK.

1. fibrillation
3. cardiac
5. ventricular

2. arteriosclerotic OR atherosclerotic
4. arteriosclerotic OR atherosclerotic
6. vascular

III. FILL IN THE BLANK.

1. arteriosclerotic coronary artery disease OR atherosclerotic coronary artery disease
3. atrioventricular
5. arteriosclerotic heart disease OR atherosclerotic heart disease

2. arteriosclerotic cardiovascular disease OR atherosclerotic cardiovascular disease
4. atrial fibrillation
6. advanced cardiac life support

Cardiology – Lesson 2

II. FILL IN THE BLANK.

1. fem
3. grafting
5. electrocardio

2. artery
4. ejection
6. pop OR popliteal

III. FILL IN THE BLANK.

1. ejection fraction
3. femoral-femoral
5. electrocardiogram

2. coronary artery bypass grafting
4. femoral-popliteal

Cardiology – Lesson 3

II. FILL IN THE BLANK.

1. anterior
3. mammary
5. cava
7. coronary OR circumflex

2. left
4. inferior
6. oblique

III. FILL IN THE BLANK.

1. left circumflex artery OR left coronary artery
3. inferior vena cava
5. left anterior descending

2. left internal mammary artery
4. left anterior oblique

Cardiology – Lesson 4

II. FILL IN THE BLANK.

1. ventricular contraction
3. obtuse
5. angioplasty
7. embolism OR embolus
9. descending

2. Myocardial
4. percutaneous transluminal
6. ventricular
8. patent ductus
10. Peripheral

FILL IN THE BLANK.

1. obtuse marginal branch
3. premature ventricular contraction
5. percutaneous transluminal coronary angioplasty
7. pulmonary embolism OR pulmonary embolus

2. left ventricle OR left ventricular
4. myocardial infarction
6. patent ductus arteriosus OR posterior descending artery
8. peripheral vascular disease

Cardiology – Lesson 5

II. FILL IN THE BLANK.

1. anterior
3. ventricular
5. descending

2. coronary OR circumflex
4. vena cava
6. mesenteric

III. FILL IN THE BLANK.

1. ventricular tachycardia
3. right anterior descending
5. right anterior oblique

2. superior vena cava
4. right coronary artery OR right circumflex artery
6. superior mesenteric artery

Review: Cardiology

I. FILL IN THE BLANK.

1. ventricular
3. anterior
5. arteriosus
7. vascular
9. superior

2. tachycardia
4. vena
6. descending
8. mammary
10. myocardial

II. MATCHING.

1. C. ventricular
3. H. transluminal
5. J. circumflex
7. F. mesenteric
9. I. atherosclerotic

2. D. grafting
4. A. ejection
6. E. embolism
8. B. oblique
10. G. left

III. MULTIPLE CHOICE.

1. left ventricle
3. patent ductus arteriosus
5. femoral-popliteal
7. atrial fibrillation
9. inferior vena cava

2. obtuse marginal branch
4. peripheral vascular disease
6. arteriosclerotic coronary artery disease
8. advanced cardiac life support
10. myocardial infarction

Fetal Measurements – Lesson 1

II. FILL IN THE BLANK.

1. biparietal diameter
3. estimated fetal weight
5. head circumference

2. femur length
4. abdominal circumference

General History – Lesson 2

II. FILL IN THE BLANK.

1. gravida
2. abortion OR abortus
3. spontaneous abortion
4. para
5. therapeutic abortion

Obstetrical Terms – Lesson 3

II. FILL IN THE BLANK.

1. cesarean
2. confinement
3. intrauterine
4. retardation
5. cephalopelvic
6. estimated

Obstetrical Terms – Lesson 4

II. FILL IN THE BLANK.

1. menstrual
2. spontaneous
3. gestational
4. alpha fetoprotein
5. vaginal birth
6. rupture
7. delivery

III. FILL IN THE BLANK.

1. large for gestational age
2. cesarean section
3. last menstrual period
4. cephalopelvic disproportion
5. maternal serum alpha fetoprotein OR maternal serum alpha-fetoprotein
6. intrauterine growth retardation
7. estimated date of confinement
8. estimated gestational age
9. rupture of membranes
10. normal spontaneous vaginal delivery
11. vaginal birth after cesarean
12. labor and delivery

Gynecology Terms – Lesson 5

II. FILL IN THE BLANK.

1. inflammatory
2. salpingo
3. hysterectomy
4. vaginal OR abdominal
5. curettage

III. FILL IN THE BLANK.

1. total abdominal hysterectomy, bilateral salpingo-oophorectomy OR total abdominal hysterectomy and bilateral salpingo-oophorectomy
2. total vaginal hysterectomy
3. dilatation and curettage OR dilation and curettage
4. pelvic inflammatory disease
5. bilateral salpingo-oophorectomy

Review: OB/GYN

I. FILL IN THE BLANK.
1. circumference
2. disproportion
3. inflammatory
4. abortion
5. Estimated
6. period
7. growth
8. hysterectomy
9. Femur
10. oophorectomy

II. MULTIPLE CHOICE.
1. cephalopelvic
2. therapeutic
3. abdominal
4. confinement
5. gestational
6. cesarean
7. alpha
8. femur
9. estimated
10. head

III. MATCHING.
1. D. spontaneous
2. C. gravida
3. A. diameter
4. B. membrane
5. F. dilatation
6. I. para
7. H. vaginal
8. J. inflammatory
9. G. delivery
10. E. intrauterine

Orthopedics – Lesson 1

II. FILL IN THE BLANK.
1. clavicular
2. cruciate
3. cervical
4. carpo
5. interphalangeal
6. orthosis OR orthotic
7. degenerative

III. FILL IN THE BLANK.
1. distal interphalangeal
2. acromioclavicular
3. carpometacarpal
4. cervical spine
5. anterior cruciate ligament
6. ankle-foot orthosis OR ankle-foot orthotic
7. degenerative disc disease

Orthopedics – Lesson 2

II. FILL IN THE BLANK.
1. iliotibial
2. metacarpo (or inter) OR inter (or metacarpo)
3. sacral
4. phalangeal
5. lumbar OR lumbosacral
6. collateral

III. FILL IN THE BLANK.
1. metacarpophalangeal
2. lumbar spine
3. interphalangeal
4. lumbosacral
5. iliotibial
6. medial collateral ligament

Orthopedics – Lesson 3

II. FILL IN THE BLANK.

1. posterior
2. temporo
3. Sacro
4. thoracic OR T-
5. proximal
6. metatarso
7. fibular

III. FILL IN THE BLANK.

1. metatarsophalangeal
2. sacroiliac
3. thoracic spine
4. temporomandibular joint
5. posterior cruciate ligament
6. proximal interphalangeal
7. tibial-fibular OR tibiofibular

Review: Orthopedics

I. FILL IN THE BLANK.

1. fibular
2. clavicular
3. disc
4. sacral
5. Carpometa
6. tibial
7. collateral
8. orthosis
9. cruciate
10. interphalangeal

II. MATCHING.

1. D. sacro
2. C. phalangeal
3. A. temporomandibular
4. G. lumbar
5. C. phalangeal
6. B. cruciate ligament
7. H. interphalangeal
8. F. cervical
9. C. phalangeal
10. I. thoracic

III. MULTIPLE CHOICE.

1. ankle-foot orthosis
2. distal interphalangeal
3. lumbosacral
4. acromioclavicular
5. degenerative disc disease
6. posterior cruciate ligament
7. iliotibial
8. temporomandibular joint
9. proximal interphalangeal
10. carpometacarpal

Radiology – Lesson 1

II. FILL IN THE BLANK.

1. posterior
2. encephalogram
3. gastrointestinal OR GI
4. Computed
5. cholangiopancreatography
6. Barium

III. FILL IN THE BLANK.

1. endoscopic retrograde cholangiopancreatography
2. barium enema
3. computed tomography
4. electroencephalogram
5. gastrointestinal
6. anteroposterior/posteroanterior

Radiology – Lesson 2

II. FILL IN THE BLANK.
1. hydroxyiminodiacetic
2. Intravenous
3. kidneys
4. bladder
5. gated acquisition
6. Magnetic
7. cholecystogram
8. cystourethrogram

III. FILL IN THE BLANK.
1. multiple gated acquisition
2. intravenous pyelogram
3. magnetic resonance imaging
4. hydroxyiminodiacetic acid OR hydroxy-iminodiacetic acid
5. kidneys, ureters, bladder
6. voiding cystourethrogram
7. oral cholecystogram

Review: Radiology

I. FILL IN THE BLANK.
1. posterior
2. Oral
3. gated acquisition
4. retrograde cholangiopancreatography
5. gastrointestinal
6. Electro
7. ureters
8. Computed
9. Voiding
10. Magnetic
11. imaging
12. iminodiacetic
13. pyelogram
14. enema

II. MULTIPLE CHOICE.
1. electroencephalogram
2. barium enema
3. posteroanterior
4. intravenous pyelogram
5. magnetic resonance imaging
6. gastrointestinal
7. computed tomography
8. kidneys, ureters, bladder
9. oral cholecystogram
10. multiple gated acquisition

Surgery – Lesson 1

II. FILL IN THE BLANK.
1. amputation
2. tunnel
3. esophagogastroduodenoscopy
4. Estimated
5. knee

III. FILL IN THE BLANK.
1. estimated blood loss
2. above-knee amputation
3. below-knee amputation
4. carpal tunnel release
5. esophagogastroduodenoscopy

Surgery – Lesson 2

II. FILL IN THE BLANK.
1. intra
2. muscular OR venous
3. endotracheal
4. jugular
5. incision
6. drainage

1. intravenous
2. endotracheal
3. intramuscular
4. incision and drainage
5. internal jugular

Surgery – Lesson 3

II. FILL IN THE BLANK.

1. reduction
2. fixation
3. nasogastric
4. Kirschner
5. laparoscopic
6. Ringer's

III. FILL IN THE BLANK.

1. nasogastric
2. open reduction, internal fixation
3. lactated Ringer's
4. Kirschner wire
5. laparotomy OR laparoscopic

Surgery – Lesson 4

II. FILL IN THE BLANK.

1. arthroplasty
2. Transurethral
3. Swan-Ganz
4. resection
5. hip OR knee
6. adenoidectomy

III. FILL IN THE BLANK.

1. total hip arthroplasty
2. transurethral resection of the bladder tumor
3. Swan-Ganz
4. total knee arthroplasty
5. transurethral resection of the prostate
6. tonsillectomy and adenoidectomy

Review: Surgery

I. FILL IN THE BLANK.

1. drainage
2. Ganz
3. amputation
4. Below
5. tracheal
6. Estimated
7. arthroplasty
8. Kirschner
9. intra
10. venous

II. MATCHING.

1. E. total
2. B. transurethral
3. H. gastric
4. A. tonsillectomy
5. G. reduction
6. D. muscular
7. F. incision
8. C. duodenoscopy
9. I. tumor
10. J. laparotomy

Ancillary Abbreviations – Lesson 1

II. FILL IN THE BLANK.

1. against
2. advice
3. Dietetic
4. activities
5. Arteriovenous
6. Cardiopulmonary
7. lymphocytic
8. acetylsalicylic
9. positive airway

III. FILL IN THE BLANK.

1. against medical advice OR American Medical Association
2. cardiopulmonary resuscitation
3. American Dietetic Association
4. arteriovenous malformation
5. activities of daily living
6. acetylsalicylic acid
7. chronic lymphocytic leukemia

Ancillary Abbreviations – Lesson 2

II. FILL IN THE BLANK.

1. extracorporeal
2. lithotripsy
3. discontinued
4. RESUSCITATE
5. birth
6. delirium

III. FILL IN THE BLANK.

1. delirium tremens
2. DO NOT RESUSCITATE
3. discontinue or discharge OR discharge or discontinue
4. date of birth
5. extracorporeal shock-wave lithotripsy

Ancillary Abbreviations – Lesson 3

II. FILL IN THE BLANK.

1. History
2. gastroesophageal
3. hydrochlorothiazide
4. physical

III. FILL IN THE BLANK.

1. history of present illness
2. gastroesophageal
3. hydrochlorothiazide
4. history and physical

Ancillary Abbreviations – Lesson 4

II. FILL IN THE BLANK.

1. dose inhaler
2. thrombocytopenic
3. no known drug
4. consciousness
5. lower lobe
6. intraocular

III. FILL IN THE BLANK.

1. loss of consciousness
2. intraocular lens
3. no known drug allergies
4. left lower lobe
5. metered dose inhaler
6. idiopathic thrombocytopenic purpura

Ancillary Abbreviations – Lesson 5

II. FILL IN THE BLANK.

1. subcutaneously (subq) OR subcutaneously
2. parenteral
3. shortness
4. nothing
5. paroxysmal
6. dyspnea
7. fenfluramine

1. nothing by mouth
2. shortness of breath
3. total parenteral nutrition
4. subcutaneous, subcutaneously OR subcutaneously
5. paroxysmal nocturnal dyspnea
6. phentermine-fenfluramine OR phentermine and fenfluramine

Review: Ancillary Abbreviations

I. FILL IN THE BLANK.
1. advice
2. Metered
3. birth
4. parenteral nutrition
5. Activities
6. Left lower
7. consciousness
8. Shortness
9. resuscitation
10. continue

II. MATCHING.
1. E. paroxysmal
2. J. allergies
3. B. tremens
4. C. airway
5. A. lymphocytic
6. H. extracorporeal
7. F. chlorothiazide
8. I. illness
9. D. acetylsalicylic
10. G. ocular

III. MULTIPLE CHOICE.
1. Dietetic
2. arteriovenous
3. purpura
4. lymphocytic
5. breath
6. metered
7. living
8. discontinue
9. lobe
10. parenteral

Review: Abbreviations

I. MULTIPLE CHOICE.
1. invalid
2. valid
3. invalid
4. invalid
5. valid
6. valid
7. invalid
8. invalid
9. invalid
10. valid

II. MULTIPLE CHOICE.
1. confinement
2. prostate
3. infarction
4. vertebral
5. inferior
6. pulmonary
7. posterior
8. salpingo-oophorectomy
9. rupture
10. congestive
11. diameter
12. proximal
13. internal
14. cystourethrogram
15. left
16. syncytial
17. ureters
18. accident
19. drainage
20. upper

III. MATCHING.

1. G. abdominal
3. A. percutaneous
5. C. clavicular
7. B. thrombosis
9. H. attack

2. J. intrauterine
4. I. fraction
6. F. living
8. D. joint
10. D. joint

IV. MULTIPLE CHOICE.

1. dilatation and curettage
3. total knee arthroplasty
5. cardiopulmonary resuscitation
7. systemic lupus erythematosus
9. patent ductus arteriosus

2. nasogastric
4. operating room
6. premature ventricular contraction
8. pulmonary embolism
10. myocardial infarction

Plurals

Plurals – Rules 1—3

I. FILL IN THE BLANK.

1. searches
3. avulsions
5. calcifications
7. cytologies
9. emergencies
11. duties
13. bosses
15. angiographies
17. leukocytes
19. peduncles

2. histories
4. extremities
6. churches
8. days
10. fractures
12. traumas
14. blushes
16. echoes
18. stitches
20. theologies

Plurals – Rule 4

I. FILL IN THE BLANK.

1. acetabula
3. brachia
5. cava
7. coccidia
9. diverticula
11. endometria
13. epithelia
15. haustra
17. infundibula
19. labia
21. mediastina
23. ostia
25. pudenda
27. rostra
29. spectra

2. antra
4. capitula
6. cilia
8. crania
10. dorsa
12. endothelia
14. frenula
16. hila
18. ischia
20. labra
22. omenta
24. plana
26. retinacula
28. spatia
30. specula

31. strata
33. tentoria
35. reticula

32. tegmenta
34. tubercula

Plurals – Rule 5

I. FILL IN THE BLANK.

1. adnexa
3. fasciae
5. trochleae
7. medullae
9. condylomata
11. valleculae
13. synechiae
15. portae
17. striae
19. genitalia
21. bullae
23. areolae
25. sellae
27. vesiculae
29. conchae

2. uvulae
4. stomata
6. vaginae
8. vertebrae
10. petechiae
12. ampullae
14. plicae
16. leiomyomata
18. linguae
20. sequelae
22. scatomata
24. conjunctivae
26. stromata
28. aurae
30. sclerae

Plurals – Rule 6

I. FILL IN THE BLANK.

1. stimuli
3. annuli
5. malleoli
7. meatus
9. humeri
11. crura
13. globi
15. vagi
17. corpora
19. thrombi
21. nevi
23. plexus
25. calculi
27. bacilli
29. villi

2. alveoli
4. viscera
6. rami
8. trunci
10. panniculi
12. glomeruli
14. limbi
16. uteri
18. menisci
20. fundi
22. canaliculi
24. bronchi
26. sulci
28. tali
30. tophi

Plurals – Rules 7—8

I. FILL IN THE BLANK.

1. ankyloses
3. irides
5. epiphyses
7. arthritides
9. pubes
11. diaphyses
13. cuspides
15. aponeuroses

2. testes
4. paralyses
6. diureses
8. prostheses
10. anastomoses
12. metastases
14. synchondroses

Plurals – Rule 9

I. FILL IN THE BLANK.

1. appendices
2. vortices
3. cruces
4. larynges
5. calices
6. thoraces
7. indices
8. falces
9. apices
10. matrices
11. cicatrices
12. phalanges
13. varices
14. cervices
15. vertices

Review: Plurals

I. FILL IN THE BLANK.

1. bronchi
2. echoes
3. labra
4. tori
5. adnexa
6. lamellae
7. appendices
8. viscera
9. branches
10. reticula
11. corpora
12. tegmenta
13. mammae
14. condylomata
15. chemistries
16. fistulae
17. falces
18. arthritides
19. panniculi
20. cicatrices
21. metaphyses
22. maxillae
23. meatus
24. foramina
25. specula
26. irides
27. humeri
28. cervices
29. lumina
30. spectra
31. apophyses
32. sulci
33. phalanges
34. malleoli
35. pelves
36. rami
37. plexus
38. synechiae
39. prostheses
40. babies

Foreign Terms

Foreign Terms – Lesson 1

II. FILL IN THE BLANK.

1. cafe au lait
2. auris dextra
3. addendum
4. cul-de-sac
5. auris sinistra
6. ad libitum
7. coup
8. aures utrae
9. bruit(s) OR bruit

Foreign Terms – Lesson 2

II. FILL IN THE BLANK.

1. Gilbert disease
2. en masse
3. in situ
4. in toto
5. en bloc
6. in ano
7. in extremis

Foreign Terms – Lesson 3

II. FILL IN THE BLANK.

1. per
2. statim
3. peau d'orange
4. raphe
5. Virchow-Robin spaces
6. status quo
7. oculus dexter
8. oculus sinister
9. Raynaud phenomenon OR Raynaud disease
10. oculus uterque

Foreign Terms – Lesson 4

II. FILL IN THE BLANK.

1. hour
2. twice a day OR twice daily
3. by mouth
4. at bedtime OR hour of sleep
5. before food
6. day
7. a drop
8. in the morning

Foreign Terms – Lesson 5

II. FILL IN THE BLANK.

1. afternoon OR betwee noon and midnight
2. three times a day OR 3 times a day
3. as needed
4. four times a day OR 4 times a day
5. every two hours OR every 2 hours
6. every day
7. every hour
8. every

Review: Foreign Terms

I. MATCHING.

1. D. in situ
2. F. stat
3. J. bruit
4. A. p.o. (per os)
5. S. ad lib
6. G. a.c.
7. E. per
8. M. q.d.
9. K. h.s.
10. I. OU
11. Q. en bloc
12. P. addendum
13. C. t.i.d.
14. L. AS
15. H. b.i.d.
16. O. status quo
17. B. in extremis
18. T. q.6 h.
19. N. cul-de-sac
20. R. en masse

Slang and Jargon

Slang and Jargon – Lesson 1

II. MATCHING.

1. F. catheter or catheterization
2. D. atrial fibrillation
3. G. appendectomy or appendicitis
4. B. chemotherapy
5. I. alkaline phosphatase
6. A. cholecystectomy
7. H. bilirubin
8. J. capsules
9. C. complete blood count with differential
10. E. bicarbonate

Slang and Jargon – Lesson 2

II. MATCHING.

1. E. detoxification
2. D. eosinophils
3. H. examination
4. A. flexible sigmoidoscopy
5. J. echocardiogram
6. I. discontinue or discharge
7. C. digoxin or digitalis
8. F. JJ stent
9. B. dipyridamole sestamibi
10. G. hematocrit

Slang and Jargon – Lesson 3

II. MATCHING.

1. C. hepatitis
2. E. Foley catheter
3. H. electrolytes
4. A. laceration
5. J. magnesium
6. G. potassium chloride
7. D. hematology and oncology
8. I. lymphocytes
9. B. potassium
10. F. hydrochlorothiazide

Slang and Jargon – Lesson 4

II. MATCHING.

1. G. oxygen saturation
2. H. milligrams
3. A. pathology
4. B. nebulizers
5. I. neuropsychiatric
6. C. medications
7. D. micrograms
8. E. metastases
9. J. neurology or neurological
10. F. monocytes

Slang and Jargon – Lesson 5

II. MATCHING.

1. H. rehabilitation
2. F. pulse oximetry
3. B. psychology/psychiatry
4. A. preoperative
5. E. saturation
6. G. prepared
7. C. postoperative
8. D. regurgitation
9. I. perforation

Slang and Jargon – Lesson 6

II. MATCHING.

1. D. ventricular tachycardia
2. F. vocational rehabilitation
3. A. sedimentation rate
4. E. segmented neutrophils
5. G. tablets
6. C. abdominal aortic aneurysm
7. B. total bilirubin

Review: Slang and Jargon

I. FILL IN THE BLANK.

1. capsules
2. flexible sigmoidoscopy
3. nebulizers
4. oxygen saturation
5. prepared
6. digoxin OR digitalis
7. appendectomy
8. atrial fibrillation
9. metastases OR metastasis
10. catheterization OR catheter

II. FILL IN THE BLANK.

1. hematocrit
2. bicarbonate
3. examination
4. milligrams
5. laceration
6. magnesium
7. perforation
8. micrograms
9. regurgitation
10. vocational rehabilitation